No Lotus Garden

Gren Wedderburn

No Lotus Garden

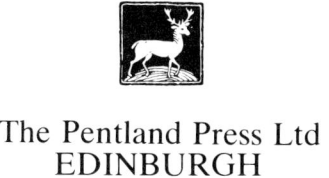

The Pentland Press Ltd
EDINBURGH

© Gren Wedderburn 1987

First published in 1987 by
The Pentland Press Ltd
Kippielaw, by Haddington
East Lothian, Scotland

Printed and bound in Scotland
by D & J Croal Ltd., Haddington.

ISBN 0 946270 37 6

To my wife Jean
who has had a lot to put up with.

Acknowledgements

The author and the publisher would like to thank the following for their help: Mrs Kaia Bell for supplying the Norwegian phrases; Miss Setsuko Wakai for checking the Japanese names and phrases; Mr A. E. V. Brown, Mr R. M. Partridge, John Swire and Sons Ltd., and the *Illustrated London News* for some of the photographs.

Contents

Foreword

I am honoured to be asked to write a foreword to this book.

I didn't know Gren during his days in China, but I remember well how the British and Commonwealth community in Japan welcomed him with open arms as, until his arrival, there was a singular lack of friendly medics there.

Until the outbreak of the Korean War, the occupation of Japan was a strict regime. There was a wide gap between the nationals of the Allied powers and the Japanese themselves, and in those early days one would not have dreamt of going to a Japanese doctor. Indeed, if one had done so, it would have been to find a Japanese clinic entirely without either modern drugs or equipment.

Although it is hard to remember now, the Japanese economy at the end of the 1940s was in a sorry state. The yen was an entirely domestic currency, continually falling in value. The Korean War changed all that. With the Americans desperate to have a secure military base, a hasty peace treaty was signed in San Francisco in 1951 and Japan took off on the economic miracle we know today.

But Gren was more than a surgeon and a family physician. He and Jean were the most generous of hosts and their house was a refuge for many.

I can well understand how Dermot Nolan wondered who Gren was, as described in the chapter "The Man Who Came to Dinner". I should know, as the "man", Paul, is now my brother-in-law.

If I was stranded in Tokyo after a late party (I lived in Yokohama at the time), Paul would insist that I come back and sleep at the Wedderburns'. "Do you think they'll mind?" I would ask. "Certainly not," Paul would reply proprietorially, adding that indeed they would be offended if I did not.

With their three daughters in addition to house guests Paul and Paddy, there was not exactly an over-supply of spare bedrooms and I seem to remember being generally housed in a sort of cupboard. But, may I say, a very comfortable cupboard.

At breakfast Jean would mildly suggest we might try and get in earlier next time, but there was never a suggestion that I was not entirely welcome.

I know many of the people in Gren's book and mention of them brings back happy memories. There were the incredibly fertile Ryans; the Duncan Frasers, now sadly parted; and above all, perhaps, that dentist *par excellence*, John Besford. Like Gren, I also had a wisdom tooth extracted by John who, in the middle of the exercise, told me it was more difficult than he had envisaged and he thought he would have to cut a hole in my cheek and pull it out that way. I was so numb with terror at the time that for a moment I belived him.

But this book is not of my reminiscences and I must allow you to read on and share Gren's love of life as manifested by him in this volume. Suffice to say that in Hong Kong Gren and Jean have not changed. They are still surrounded by friends; both still do many good works without thought of or wish for publicity; in addition, Gren is always ready to share with you his tips for the races. On this last point may I, as the keeper of many people's overdrafts, suggest that you will do well to ignore them.

Sir Michael Sandberg.

Preface or A word in advance

This book is my account of my boyhood in China and later life as a surgeon in China and Japan just after the Second World War. I have tried to keep out details which are not directly related to those times. In this preface I would like to take the opportunity of filling in a few of the background details.

My surname, Wedderburn, is an old Scottish name; in fact the National Standard Bearer of Scotland, Lord Dundee, is a Wedderburn.

My grandfather was a Minister in the parish of Madderty in Perthshire. My father graduated in Divinity at Edinburgh University. His elder brother became Governor of the Colony of Ceylon and his younger brother, an officer in the Cameronians, a Scottish regiment, was killed in World War I and buried at Bois Grenier just before I was born. I was named Grenier after him and have spent a lot of time explaining how I received this name ever since.

My father became a missionary of the Church of Scotland in Manchuria in 1910. He married Susan Crooks, who was a nurse with the Church of Ireland Mission in China.

My elder brother, my sister and I went to school at the China Inland Mission School at Chefoo, one of the old Treaty Ports in North China. In my teens my brother and I were sent to George Watson's College in Edinburgh. As missionaries had furlough only once every five years, my parents left me in Scotland as a young schoolboy and next saw me as a medical student. My brother Laurie and I stayed in a school boarding house; during the holidays we presented ourselves at the abodes of relations. One grand-uncle and two grand-aunts liked me and detested my brother. Another grand-aunt considered me to be lacking in all human virtues and likeable characteristics, but thought Laurie was an intelligent sort of saint. The two of us knew where to go for holidays and seldom met except at the house of three maiden aunts at Larne in Northern Ireland. Fortunately, our Irish aunts seemed to like us both.

I graduated from Edinburgh University in 1938. When World War II started I tried to join the Royal Air Force, expecting to be called up in a few weeks. The weeks stretched out, so it was necessary to try to find some temporary employment. I visited an office in search of a post which I considered suitable to my talents but I was rejected. Descending the steps onto the street, I encountered a girl whom I had known slightly as a student. She was walking along supporting her cheek with one hand, as she had just left a dentist's office. Her name was Jean McEwan. As we were both suffering minor setbacks, our common misfortune forged a bond which resulted in our getting married a year later.

I consider myself fortunate that for the six years that I served in the RAF as a medical officer my postings were with Fighter Command. I joined 257 Squadron in the latter half of the Battle of Britain and stayed with the squadron for nearly a year. The Commanding Officer was R. R. Stanford Tuck, at that time the leading fighter pilot. Fighter Command was relatively small and at one time or another I met most of those who were famous. The great compliment paid to these men in Churchill's immortal phrase was justified beyond measure.

In 1942 I was posted to India, and again considered myself lucky to be with Fighter Units except for a thoroughly enjoyable nine months with 353 Squadron in Delhi. 353 were the only Transport Squadron then in India. As Medical Officer the opportunity to fly to the major cities as well as to some less desirable places was fully utilised. For the rest of the three years I was at jungle air-strips on the Indo-Burmese border; when I became Wing Medical Officer, some of the strips were in India and others a mile or two away were over the border in Burma. The Wing moved forward by easy stages into Burma and reached Rangoon the day after it was captured in May 1945. Hygiene and sanitation occupied a great deal of the time of a medical officer in the jungle and I became a leading authority on the construction of latrines; subsequently this knowledge does not seem to have been of any particular benefit.

After demobilisation I decided to seek the advice of Sir James R. Learmonth, Professor of Surgery of the Medical School in Edinburgh. I was proceeding to this office when we encountered each other in the courtyard.

He asked my why I was there and listened to my story.

"Report to Wards 7 and 8 tomorrow morning at 8.30. Ask the sister to give you a white coat."

Sir James nodded as he turned towards the professorial block.

My fate was decided.

Chapter 1

A BOYHOOD IN CHINA

By cart to Chefoo School — Poling along the Sungari — Warmth at the inns — Horse-dealers and skulduggery.

My father, who was a missionary, was fond of saying that there were two types of missionary: the statesmen and the coolies. The statesmen with the Church of Scotland mission ran the administration and tried to convert the people. They lived in the comparative comfort of Mukden, the capital of Manchuria. The coolies lived far away from their colleagues, and were in charge of districts the size of Belgium.

The town we lived in was Chao Yang Chun, over a hundred miles east from the railway towards the Korean border. The line joined Harbin in northern Manchuria, and ran through Mukden to Dairen on the peninsula at the south which jutted into the Gulf of Pichili.

Our house with its large garden was enclosed by a high wall. A door led through the wall opposite the house into a second enclosed compound where the coachman or carter lived beside the stable and cart shed. Two large doors opening onto the street formed the gate through which the cart could go; one half of the door had a small postern for pedestrian use.

Ten yards outside the gate was a facing strip of wall which forced a cart to turn sharply left or right to pass the ends of the wall. This was to hinder devils who, as everyone knows, cannot turn corners. All over Manchuria every house large enough to have a wall and gate had such a wall hiding the gate from view and acting as a barrier against devils. When our carter ploughed the garden, the furrows were made in graceful curves, and so it was with every furrow in every field in the country. The curve made it tough going for the devils trying to damage or steal the farmer's crop. Dragons, on the other hand, were more fortunate, since they could easily negotiate turns.

During the Manchurian winter, snow blankets the ground from November till March. The ground becomes frozen for four to five feet down and the thermometer plunges to minus thirty to forty Celsius. Double windows were fitted onto our house in the autumn; in the corner of each room stood a tall round iron stove. The fire in the stove was lit in autumn and stayed alight till spring, glowing almost red-hot.

Fortunately there was an anthracite surface mine not far from Chao Yang Chun, but it was wise to stock up a winter's supply in the huge coal shed behind the kitchen.

Although I do not think that I was ever in Chao in summer after I was seven years of age, I have many memories of the short, hot summers with days of blistering sun, punctuated by spells of heavy rain or by fierce dust storms when the dry west winds blew from across Mongolia and the Gobi desert.

At the age of seven I was sent to school in Chefoo in Shantung province. The Chinese characters for China are the two characters for "middle" and "kingdom". The kingdom is within the Great Wall comprising the true China; outside the wall lies the land of barbarians. China today includes Tibet, Mongolia and Manchuria, but the true China is really the land of its exact original culture. Chefoo is definitely south of the Great Wall and part of the Middle Kingdom.

Mainly because of the terrible winter, Chefoo school surrendered its pupils for a two month winter holiday, a short Easter holiday, and a one month summer holiday. In winter our journey from Chao Yang Chun to school took at least a week. In summer, by the time one got home one would have to leave the next day to be back in time for the new term, because the road from the railway to Chao became a sea of mud. The lead horse could eaisly be drowned in the mud. Some days one would progress only four or five miles. My father and mother would come to stay in Chefoo for the summer or we would travel the short distance from school to Pei Tei Ho, a resort on the coast connected by rail to Peking.

During the winter, when the roads were frozen, the journey by cart from Chao to Teihling on the railway took four days. Two hours by train landed us in Mukden. We stayed in Mukden a day to join the school party of some dozen or more pupils. The party travelled overnight by rail to Dairen to board the somewhat dilapidated SS *Yung Lee* for a further twenty-four hour sea-trip to Chefoo.

The party of children was looked after by an escort, either a missionary or a businessman. The missionary would try to achieve reasonable behaviour from his treasures by appealing to our Christian upbringing. The businessman adopted a more pragmatic approach — outright bribery — in an effort to prevent the little brutes from committing more than the normal quota of misdemeanours. He resorted to handing out candies, ice cream, and soft drinks as a practically uninterrupted process.

There was little doubt which type was the more popular.

Other children sailed to the school at Chefoo and Shanghai. Eddy Brown, now with Swire Ltd. of Hong Kong, was with the Chefoo School party on a Butterfield and Swire ship in the early thirties. While they were at sea, the ship was taken by pirates, and held for three days. The crew and passengers endured ill-treatment, but the thirty-odd children had the run of the ship and the time of their lives.

Before I went to school we did travel in summer but we used the river, called the Huang Fu, which flowed a mile or so from Chao Yang Chun. My father usually bought a large sampan together with its crew. A small stuffy cabin was situated aft with a forward cubby hole for the crew. The Huang Fu was a lazy, muddy stream with sand banks on which the sampan frequently grounded. The crew of three boatmen spent many hours a day with a long bamboo pole over which they would bend, resting one end of the pole on the river bed and the other against a shoulder. Leaning on the pole they would thrust and shove as they walked from the bow to the stern, pushing the sampan along or fending it off the sand banks, then walk back to the prow and start again. This slow progress went on for three days but excitement rose as the sampan approached the Sungari[1] which flowed swiftly with clear water from the melting snows.

On the Sungari the poling stopped, the current being enough to whisk the boat along. There were two or three rapids where the water rushed at breakneck speed, smashing against huge rocks in mid-stream. Before the rapids, the crew hauled the boat alongside a village pier to take on a pilot. The pilot was one of the senior villagers who had graduated to his position after a long apprenticeship, for the village made its living from the rapids and the villagers were skilful. The pilot knew the river in all its moods from the time the ice melted, as it gradually rose and swelled in ferocity,

---

[1] The Sungari River has now been dammed just south of Kirin, creating an enormous reservoir.

until the full flow of summer slowly diminished towards autumn and the ice returned. The pilot, a master of his art, manned a steering oar while the crew worked like demons to keep some headway as the boat hurtled down between rocks with the water seething, here with menacing smoothness, and there turbulent, broken, smashing against emergent jagged rocks or foaming over hidden boulders. My mother sat on the cabin roof, her feet braced against the deck, clutching me in a tight embrace, full of fear; but a boy loved it and so did my father.

We never went upstream, but many junks did, and this was the village's source of income. Three villagers had long poles to sheer off rocks while the pilot manned a huge steering oar astern. If the boat were small and unladen, five men on the bank pulled on the rope to move the boat upstream in the calmer waters near the bank. A heavily laden junk needed a mixture of stout-hearted men and tough young women, plus a singer. Each person held his or her individual rope, leaning forward with the rope passing over a pad on their shoulder and attached by a pattern of reins to the main tow-rope. Taking the pull they bent against the strain. The pilot used hand signals to the singer, who started to chant; the gang worked as one man, heaving and singing together. The singer paced slowly backward with his eye on the pilot. My father told me that the pitch of his song conveyed his order to the mass of straining humanity.

If a man lurched or faltered he would use a trip device to disconnect his strain rope, twisting out of line so that others would not stumble over him and thus alter the total rhythm of the steady, pulsating, twenty manpower strain on the tow-rope.

It was bitter work, probably the most sustained continuous hard work accomplished anywhere in the world, but, like all Chinese, they were proud of their skill and strength. It was team work of the highest order and their labours did not come cheap.

Once my father took me along behind the team, well clear of the tow-rope, right up along the whole length of a rapid. At the top they rested, sitting down to eat dumplings, and were delighted to see, possibly for the first time in their lives, a foreign child. They offered me choice pieces of food, reached out in wonder to touch my fair skin, patted me, and had animated conversations with my father.

"Is he betrothed?" they asked. All rich men's sons were betrothed from early childhood. A missionary was a poor man by our standards but by theirs we must have been as rich as Croesus.

When we reached Kirin my father sold the boat, usually with a small profit. From Kirin there was a branch line to the main railway, but the trip was not without danger.

Once, when I was too young to remember, we were attacked by a robber band who relieved my father of all his cash and my mother of her wedding ring. Because my father did not have much cash, the chief brandished an enormous sword, believing that there must be a hidden hoard of money. As the crew were beaten with long staves, my mother watched with horror, sure that my father would come in for the same treatment. Her horror mounted as the robber chief, still holding his sword, lifted me up in front of him, held me there, laughed, put his hand in his pocket and handed me half a dollar.

My brother Laurie was about five at the time. He went up to the robber chief and reached up his hand to the robber's liberal paunch.

"Ooh, what a fat man," he remarked in Chinese.

The robbers howled with mirth. Chinese have a great respect for fat men and the chief himself was delighted.

My mother gave up wearing a wedding ring after the third disappeared under similar circumstances.

My most vivid memories are of the journeys to school. A mountain of blankets covered the flat surface of the cart, my brother and I were well tucked in, our fur hats exposing only our eyes and mouths.

The cold was intense. If we fell asleep, father kept an eye on us in case our noses were frostbitten. On waking it was necessary to rub our eyes with a glove to release the eyelashes frozen together.

One horse was in the shafts, while the leader was ahead on reins. The carter sat on the left-hand shaft and my father in the cart or on the right-hand shaft, from which he could jump down and walk. At mid-day and in the evening we stopped at an inn, deserted at lunchtime but full by the evening.

The main export product of Manchuria was the soya bean. This rich harvest could not be moved until the roads froze and the big, flat, two-wheeled carts could set off, covered with a huge mound of sacks, on the journey to the railroad. They travelled in convoys, partly for protection from robbers, but also for mutual assistance. One large pony pulled in the shafts, with two ponies in the line ahead and a front rank of four abreast. Of the seven or so animals, about three would be mules. The horses pulled well early in the day but the stamina of the mules was greater, and by early afternoon the mules were doing most of the work. Nearly all the carts had this mixture. When a steep hill was reached, one team of horses would be hitched in front in addition to a regular team. The two carters would yell at the fifteen odd animals, the crack of their whips sounded like pistol shots in the frosty air, while steam rose from the straining horses. The carters were dexterous with the whip attached to the end of a short bamboo; they could flick a fly from the ear of a mule in the front rank or administer a vicious cut on the hide of a recalcitrant animal.

The carters were tough and ribald, and even the ordinary Chinese, no laggards with bad language, admired their swearing. The carters took great care of their animals, hitching up the teams at about three a.m. in the most awful cold, to get away by four. At about ten the convoy pulled into an inn, and the teams were unshackled and fed from troughs. The carter then had his first meal of the day. They were off again by eleven, stopping for the day by three in the afternoon. The carter fed the animals again and tethered them before he had his evening meal and went to sleep. He was up again to feed them at midnight before snatching another two hours' sleep before starting another day. If an animal was not fit it might be allowed to walk on a rope behind or even be left at the inn until the cart came back.

Occasionally a gruesome relic might be left behind. As the carts had no brakes and when loaded weighed over a ton, going downhill could be a hazardous business on roads with snow so packed that it had become ice. Various strategems were adopted. Two or three animals might be harnessed to the rear of the cart facing downhill; goaded by the whiplash they strained against the weight of the cart, struggled and heaved but were slowly drawn backward step by step. Another method was to ram a stout pole between the wheel spokes so that the pole engaged against the platform of the cart, effectively locking the wheel; a second pole was thrust just in front of the first free spoke so that when the first pole was withdrawn the wheel whirled round until in a fraction of a second the second pole engaged against the platform. Even with the wheels locked the cart might slide for a yard or two. With a succession of loaded carts, with many animals and carters involved, accidents happened. A wheel passing over a leg fractured the bones and if it passed over the body death was imminent. Occasionally a wooden coffin knocked up by a local carpenter lay by the roadside. The carter left his comrade's body, frozen stiff in its coffin, to be picked up on the return trip and taken back home. No one was going to dig a grave in ground frozen solid for six feet deep. Even in the spring it took time for the ground to thaw out from the surface so that the graves were shallow and the earth piled on top of and around the coffin. Grave mounds were a common sight at the end of the winter; although the majority were buried deeper after a month, some graves remained as permanent mounds at the side of a field.

Before setting off on our journey my mother provided a variety of cooked food, pies, meat loaf, jellies and cake. Chinese food, provided it was cooked and piping hot, we judged to be safe to eat. Frequently we ate the food provided by the inn especially if rice was available; rice was something of a luxury in Manchuria. There was a basic charge for the rice with extra cost added for the side dishes of pork, fish and vegetables. The bill was paid as soon as the last side dish had been delivered. The carters would give a tip of one or two cents but my father usually added ten per cent, say twenty cents. The waiter picked up the money and in a voice loud enough for everyone to hear, including the other servants, he shouted, "Thank you for the forty cents." He put the tip in a wooden box and no matter how small or large the tip he always called out double the actual amount. Everyone got a lot of "face".

Chang Tsu Lin and K'ao Tien played out a charade ending in a typical Chinese arrangement and compromise. The Chinese characters of K'ao Tien's name meant "Trust in Heaven", hardly a suitable name for a robber chief. As my parents were travelling to Chao Yeng Chun for the first time in 1913, "Trust in Heaven" with his robber band, reported as 500 strong but probably 200 or 300 men, captured Chao. Chang Tsu Lin could not allow this to persist in a town under his suzerainty, and mobilising a considerable force he advanced on the town to camp outside the walls. The result of a fight could not be in doubt as Chang had better equipped and far superior forces; still there would be bloodshed, innocent inhabitants killed and it would all be costly. Emissaries met and discussions took place so that by the end of the second day K'ao Tien was a colonel, and all the band of robbers were enrolled, en masse, into Chang's army.

My parents had halted at Hailung some twelve miles away until the position clarified. They were called to see the senior magistrate, dressed in the old Mandarin style of fine robes with flowing sleeves.

7

It was in the evening of the "cease fire". He said all the polite things and insisted on personally handing them cups of tea before reporting that all was well in Chao Yeng Chun. My father could proceed safely the next morning to his new parish.

"Trust in Heaven" and his soldiers remained for several years as the garrison.

He called on my father a day or two afterwards to say that he was in charge of this somewhat dangerous town and district but that they would be completely safe under his able protection. He became a frequent visitor. After Laurie was born he was very impressed by two things; that Laurie was fed on goat's milk and that he slept outside in his cot at midday. He considered this to be a toughening up process started in early life, responsible for the characteristics which he attributed to all foreign devils.

We got to know many of the garrison. Usually we stopped at the guardhouse over the city gate when we returned from sledging or a picnic in the hills and had a cup of tea while enjoying the excitement of playing with real guns or wielding the swords, while many of the soldiers in turn might stroke our hair in wonder. Our hair was light coloured when we were young and its soft texture was in marked contrast to the rather wiry hair of Chinese children.

Chinese cows were never milked except by their calves and my mother was at her wits' end coping with Laurie's feeding until a fellow missionary sent a nanny goat from Kirin. A few Swiss hornless goats had been imported some years before by Danes. By mixing goat's milk with water and malt the mixture became Laurie's, and after I was born my, staple diet.

The Swiss goat is somewhat more stocky than allied species; even the billy goat did not have horns and they had a generous fleece of pure white wool. We always had a billy goat with two or three nannies. They were sagacious animals full of character, mischief and charm when they cared to exhibit some charm.

The male we called Max, presuming it to be a Swiss name. Max liked nothing better than to have his neck scratched and his back rubbed. If I stopped scratching before Max was contented he was liable to butt me, often sending me flat on my back, but it was all good natured fun. The goats lived in the compound alongside the stable. My mother made the mistake, early on in their mutual acquaintance, of letting them into the garden. The goats proceeded immediately to the coloured objects, nipping off the flowers on which she had lavished care and love; they then started on the vegetables and in the absence of anything better, the bark of the trees was an acceptable alternative. When everything was frozen stiff in winter they were allowed into the garden to romp and play provided that the washing had been taken in. They would make very short shrift of a coloured sweater or jersey, before starting on the plainer pants and vests.

One cold morning my father called me over to the window. He had spotted the cook's wife making her way from the door of the garden along the path cleared of snow and flanked by the piles of snow; he had also spotted Max advancing with obvious ill intent. The cook's wife was a fat dumpy little woman, now almost round in her voluminous winter garments. Max let her pass but the sight of her ample posterior was too much for him; lowering his head, with three quick strides he gave her a goodly dunt, hurling her into a mound of snow. Max withdrew a pace or two while the woman attempted to rise. She was only half upright, presenting her large behind as a target, before Max resumed the genial task of butting her again to sprawl her once more in the snow. This time she was more circumspect rising, to keep Max in view before she walked backward some ten paces; meanwhile Max seemed to have lost all interest in the good woman until she turned around, when he sprang into action spilling her once more. My mother joined us to see what was causing the mirth. With indignation at our callous disregard for a fellow female she ordered me to intervene. I ran out along the path, dodged an attack by Max who was enjoying himself, grabbed the fleece on the back of his neck and vaulted astride him. The boy goatherd, who looked after them and loved them dearly, milked them and took them to the hills on summer afternoons, had discovered that if you sat on Max's back he became docile right away. Max would not attempt to dislodge the rider; however he would not move, stubbornly refusing to become a transport animal.

A close neighbour had feeding problems with her baby; she had been impressed with the progress made by Laurie and me so she asked if she could borrow one of the nanny goats, which was delivered by the goat boy. A few days later mother asked the boy if he had given instructions on milking, especially as only the boy could do this. He replied that he had advised on what the goat should be given for food, but had not mentioned milking.

Mother went round to see what was happening, to be told that there had been some difficulty at first while the goat was firmly held and the baby lifted up to suck from a teat. After a day or two, the goat would come into the room as soon as she heard the baby cry and lie down beside the baby who then got on with feeding. The baby started to put on weight; the feeding problem had been solved.

The entrance to an inn was through the kitchen where two big fires burned. From the kitchen a traveller went through a big door into the main hall, possibly sixty or a hundred feet long. Down the whole of each side ran a platform raised by three feet, like a railway station with the thoroughfare in the middle. The flue from the kitchen fire ran the length of the platform (called a *kang*) to its chimney at the other end. The *kang*, covered by a rush mat, was warm to the touch; one sat cross-legged at low tables on the *kang* to eat, and pushed the table aside to lay out the bedding roll.

By the time we got in, the carters were finishing their evening meal. The inns were havens of warmth and soon the lamps were dimmed. Figures lay comatose in long ranks on the *kangs*, and the air was likely to be rent by stentorian snores. There was one additional action we took: namely, to lay a line of Keating's anti-bug powder in a low rampart on the *kang* round our bedding. I do not think this impressed the bugs much, who just jumped over it. Through the night, beyond the paper covering the small windows, the sounds of two hundred odd horses were a constant background as they whinnied, stamped their shod hooves, snorted and pulled on their tethers.

My sister Diana remained in China with our parents while my brother and I went to school in Scotland. I asked her for her memories of travelling in China, and I can do no better than to quote what she wrote.

"That was the point in the day's travelling which I liked best — arriving at the inn, and the horses and mules being let out of harness and rolling on their backs. The flailing hooves were a bit alarming but I loved going into the inn, settling down on the *kang* and looking at the strings of onions and peppers hanging from the rafters.

"The coolies and carters would draw off boiling water from the cauldron in the corner and wash in it without adding any cold water to cool it down. They seemed to be able to wash in and drink scalding water. Some fellows would come in playing two spoons or sticks together and a cricket might chirp from the corner. Everyone would stare at us and make rude remarks about our 'ugly' curly hair.

"The Japanese railway was built soon after we moved the dozen miles in Hailung so we had made our last journey by cart."

To buy a horse one hired a middleman and explained to him the requirements, and he then contacted a seller. These two sat on the ground opposite each other, spread a small cloth between them and put their hands under the cover. No words were spoken but information was passed and the transaction accomplished by pressure of the fingers. Naturally the opportunities for skulduggery were beyond imagination. Horse dealers always had an unsavoury reputation, a role inherited nowadays by second-hand car dealers. At one time my father became an equine enthusiast and, fired by some fantasy, bought a Russian ex-cavalry horse, large and dapple grey.

We all turned out for the first harnessing and admired it; the carter overcame some persistent resistance by the animal before he had it harnessed between the shafts. Suddenly it bolted, lowered its head and galloped through the postern gate. Although the horse got through, the cart was crushed against the gate on either flank. Both cart and gate were demolished. The cavalry charger tore down the streets of Chao Yang Chun, knocking over hawker stalls, half obliterating a market, and creating a chaos which gave rise to a host of claims, eventually met from the funds of the Church of Scotland.

As my father rushed after the animal, the evidence of damage was apparent on all sides; he realised he would have to foot the bill, but had visions of the horse heading for the Steppes, adding up to a total loss. He ran to the mayor, who gave hasty orders, and the huge east and west gates set in Chao Yang Chun's city wall were closed. The horse eventually tired and was recaptured.

The next day my father stood behind the two horse dealers as they sat, their hands under the blanket, no flicker of expression on their faces; the cavalry charger changed ownership again at a very reduced figure. My father's distrust of horse dealers was by now absolute. Apart from practically every hawker in Chao accepting this heaven-sent opportunity to overclaim his losses, the whole affair became an enormous joke, having all the elements of slapstick comedy. The whole population of twenty thousand roared its head off.

Even Chang Tsu Lin, the famed warlord of Manchuria, heard about it. Learning that my father was at a railway station where his train had drawn in, Chang sent an aide to ask my father to corroborate the story which had not lost in the telling. Chang quite approved of missionaries for the education they gave and hospitals they set up. He backed the Mukden Medical College run by the Church of Scotland. As warlords go, Chang was a benevolent dictator and ran his province with considerable benefit to all, but a successful warlord of Manchuria who might have become Emperor of China did not fit in with Japanese plans. In 1931, as Chang was returning from a visit to Peking where the "golden dust" had been sprinkled in front of him, a gesture symbolising elevation to the monarchy, his train was blown up when crossing a bridge.

My brother and I were bumping along in the cart one cold and frosty morning when father drew our attention to the landscape on our right, which was notable only for a singular lack of features. My brother Laurie nudged me, throwing a sidelong glance to the left. On every telegraph pole, about eighteen in all, was nailed a human head. A band of robbers had been summarily dealt with and their heads, preserved by the cold, would look down on travellers for another three months till spring came. When we reached Liaoyuan with its massive forty-foot walls and cavernous gate, we saw the head, trunk and severed limbs of the robber chief on a wall: a further deterrent.

In Chao Yang Chun my father had made repeated attempts to interest one of the senior wealthy and influential men of the town in Christianity. Politely received, he was equally politely rebuffed. Immediately after the attack on Pearl Harbour in 1941, my father was arrested as a spy, condemned to death and cast into prison. His sentence was commuted and after four months he rejoined other missionaries in Mukden. He walked into the house where my mother and others were dining, emaciated, bearded, dressed only in his underclothes, and caked with filth, mud and excreta from the cell shared with a score of criminals. The people froze in horror at the sudden apparition.

"Don't you know me, Sue?" he said to my mother. "I'm Dal, your husband."

After his arrest my mother had been alone, in terrible distress. The rich man from Chao had been ushered in, with two servants to collect what goods she wished to take. He had taken her back to live in his house where he and his family had tried to comfort her and offer solace. This act was of course noted by the Japanese police; it was an act involving a great risk to himself; a typically Chinese gesture of friendship. She had stayed for a week until arrangements were made for her to go to Mukden.

A BOYHOOD IN CHINA

During World War II my mother and father were interned in Nagasaki, Japan. Father was on a hillside herding cows when the atomic bomb exploded three miles away; he was knocked over by the blast and lightly singed as though sunburnt. The Atomic Energy Commission contacted him when my parents returned to live with my sister in Australia, in order to take regular blood tests. This he regarded as a piece of nonsense. When the "sunburn" from the explosion had worn off, he felt as fit as ever. After my mother died he returned to Scotland. The Atomic Energy Commission was still hard on his heels; but they rewarded him for going to the hospital, took his blood sample, and gave him a cup of tea and ten shillings for his trouble, so it all made sense to a Scotsman. My father could hardly wait for the next three-monthly postcard to report to the hospital.

When he was in his eighties, he travelled to South Africa by ship. While descending the companionway in a rough sea, he fell and struck his head. He never regained consciousness.

Chapter 2

MY FATE IS SEALED

Edinburgh and Professor Learmonth — Peg-leg and pearls — The Subject is Shanghai.

Very few surgeons had been trained in the war years. To make up for lost time, doctors demobilised from the services were enrolled as Class One and Class Three trainees. I was one of the trainees under James Learmonth, Professor of Surgery at the Medical School in Edinburgh. The class in which we found ourselves seemed to depend on some whim of Sir James which he certainly never explained, but it made a big difference. Some of us were paid £550 a year and the others £350. Both salaries were breadline payments, but Class Three at £350 was more breadline than the other. I was fortunate to be Class One after nine months.

As a member of Class One, I had the privilege of joining the coffee session after an out-patient clinic. It was at one of these sessions that Sir James spoke to me.

"Wedderburn," he said.

"Yes, sir," I replied, somewhat startled at being singled out of the throng.

"You were born in China weren't you?"

"Yes, sir."

"Come to my office in the Research Block at four o'clock."

"Yes, sir."

Sir James was not going to shed any light on this order. There was some speculation amongst us as to what this might portend. A popular theory was that the Professor had read an article in a surgical magazine by a Chinese surgeon with which he violently disagreed, and because of the accident of my nativity the brunt of his wrath was about to fall on my head. Then again there might be no connection whatsoever between my birthplace and the reason for my presence in his office. The consensus was that I was to be confronted with some dreadful misdemeanour of general or surgical behaviour, probably both.

"What is it about?" I asked his secretary some ten minutes before the appointed time.

"Dr Burton wants to see you."

"Who is Dr Burton?"

"A friend of the Professor's. I don't know why he wants to see you. He is in there," she said, pointing to the office.

Dr Tom Burton was seated at the Professor's desk. He waved me to the chair opposite and without preliminaries he said:

"Sir James tells me that you were born in China and went to school there."

"Yes."

"Well, I am in a practice in Shanghai. We have a surgeon now, but we want a young surgeon," he said.

"I have not passed the fellowship exams yet," I replied.

"Sir James says you will."

"Oh!" I had been brought up sharp — I wished I could have shared his confidence. The interview continued and ended with my assurance that although my wife would have to be consulted, I was fairly certain she would agree to come to China with me. After the interview, Tom Burton limped out.

As he limped, a picture flashed to my mind of an incident which had occurred earlier. Sir James Learmonth had been walking up the stairs of the Royal Infirmary of Edinburgh accompanied by his two subchiefs. Immediately behind were the two clinical tutors followed by a motley crowd of Class One and Class Three doctors, sisters, interns, research scholars and one student.

At the tail-end of the retinue was a lone man, dressed in a Savile Row suit. He was the only one not in a doctor's white coat. He mounted the stairs by taking two steps with the left leg and bringing the right alongside onto the same step while leaning heavily on a stick. Sir James glanced back at the stolid figure, turned and descended through the ranks of his followers to join him, and together they climbed slowly past us all. The man with the limp and walking stick joined the ward round; he was obviously both a doctor and the Professor's friend — Dr Tom Burton.

Later I was to find out that when Tom Burton arrived in the United Kingdom a week before, he had limped heavily off a BOAC Argonaut, his artificial leg (he had lost one leg on the Somme in World War I) containing a wad of dollars well tamped down by an assortment of pearls which filled the cavity of the leg nearly to the knee joint.

He had been carrying the pearls for Jedeon Pearls Incorporated,

15

to whom was sublet the large waiting room of the downtown offices of Drs Marshall, Jackson, and Partners in Shanghai.

Jedeon had suggested to Burton, one of the partners, that as pearls were in short supply in the United Kingdom, Burton should take a consignment handily concealed in his leg. Jedeon had asked for a certain sum to be paid to him. Anything that the carrier could get above the sum was his own. He was given an address to go to in London. On the tarmac of London Airport the artificial leg had seemed to clatter with every step that Burton took, but his mission was successful. We never found out what Burton's profit was.

For a girl who had never been farther afield from the United Kingdom than on one trip to Holland, my wife Jean showed neither hesitation nor indecision. She told me to go ahead and accept. As soon as it was decently light next morning I called Dr Burton. We were coming.

Sir James was right; my efforts seemed to satisfy the examiners for the Fellowship of the Royal College of Surgeons of Edinburgh. The Ministry of Transport allocated me a berth on the MV *Anchises* of the Blue Funnel line sailing from Liverpool, and a berth for Jean and our daughter on the MV *Canton* some six months later.

It was 1947. During my last week in Edinburgh I went to watch a rugby match and there met a pilot from an RAF squadron with which I had served in India. On telling the pilot, who had reverted to his employment as policeman, that I was leaving for Shanghai, he looked at me with wonder.

"Haven't you had enough?" he asked.

Chapter 3

BACK TO CHINA

Some sly scotches at sea — Sweating it out at Port Swettenham — Arrival in Shanghai.

The freighter SS *Anchises* cast off her lines to move out into the Mersey and drop the skyline of Liverpool astern. A voyage by freighter can be enjoyable if two criteria are met — fellow passengers must be agreeable and the crew amiable. The captain considered rightly that he was in command of a vessel with the primary purpose of carrying cargo; passengers in his opinion were an unmitigated nuisance. The ship had berths for twelve passengers wished onto him by a mistaken policy of the owners. He was not, however, in any way going to alter the routine of his ship to suit the passengers. Meals were served at times convenient for the crew's watchkeeping duties. Notices abounded confining passengers to limited areas.

The owners, in their wisdom, decided that passengers must be allowed to have a drink but the bar was open for the stipulated minimum time — half an hour before lunch, and half an hour before the uncivilised hour of six for dinner. After dinner the long evening wore on till nine when the bar was opened again for one hour. Doyle, a cheerful Liverpool steward, doubled as our cabin steward and bar steward. During a conversation one morning while he was cleaning my cabin, he guardedly hinted that he did not share the captain's views either on passenger abstemiousness or on discipline. In happier times he had served on a Cunarder. Doyle made life tolerable; a few minutes before he slid down the grill of the bar at ten p.m. he would disappear for a few minutes to set three deck chairs up on the deck outside the saloon.

As he handed us our last drink he would enquire, "Two or three biscuits with your morning tea, sir?"

"Two I think tomorrow, Doyle. Thank you."

Having finished our official quota we would stroll out on deck, sit in the chairs and reach stealthily behind the chairs to grasp one of the two large whisky sodas reposing on the deck. It was necessary to maintain a sharp seamanlike lookout in case the captain hurried past on some urgent errand. Presumably there was no law forbidding us from this habit but we did not want our life-line, Doyle, to "cop it", and suffer some horrible nautical fate such as being keel-hauled or flung into irons.

We made a fast passage to Penang, stopping for only four hours to bunker at Aden. The delays started at Penang where the dock facilities, crippled by the war, were totally inadequate. The ship rode at anchor for a week before going alongside. The stevedores were also a war legacy, suffering from years of near starvation; their languid ineffectual movements were painful to watch. For once passengers and captain were united in the frustration of seeing work which should have been accomplished in two days at the most, drag out over five or six. At last we set sail for Port Swettenham, indeed aptly named.

To reach Port Swettenham a ship crawls up a creek for a couple of hours to tie up against the wharf. Across the river are miles of ghastly swamp, and the river teems with nasty-looking fish and sea snakes. Hemmed in by the jungle beyond the warehouses, an iron-ship gets steadily hotter, and even the relative cool of the night does not bring the heat of the ship back to what it had been on the previous dawn.

The next six days were a mounting prolongation of discomfort. Even a cold shower gave no relief, as the water in the ship's tanks was as hot as everything else. Eventually the captain relented, allowing cold beer for quite generous periods. Port Swettenham may now be quite a pleasant place to visit on an airconditioned ship with Kuala Lumpur only a couple of hours by taxi, but in 1947 terrorists were active in the area and the trip was not at all safe.

In Singapore things went very quickly. Four days saw us out at sea again and the contrast provided by the dock-workers at Holt's Wharf in Hong Kong was a joy to watch. The evening shift swarmed on board to start shifting cargo as though their lives depended on their efforts.

However, delays were not eliminated. The *Anchises* left the wharf to anchor in the harbour because the Shanghai river pilots had gone on strike; so Hughes, a friend made on the *Anchises*, and I transferred to the *Tsidane*, a Dutch-owned boat. The Captain was not daunted by the lack of a pilot; he declared that he would take the ship up the Whang Po to Shanghai without a pilot if necessary. On entering the ship's bar the Chinese barman informed us that his bunk adjoined the bar, and that he was ready and willing to serve at any time of the night or day. Very shortly two very attractive girls came in, cementing the opinion that our transfer was a sound move.

Hughes sat at the Chief Engineer's table for dinner; my place was at the Chief Officer's. The Engineer was a handsome, clean-cut, darkhaired Dutchman. The First Mate was a clean-cut, handsome, blond Dutchman; the Captain was a clean-cut, handsome, blond Dutchman. I picked up the menu.

"Yes," said the Chief, "you will have to order from the menu now, but better order from the Chinese chef from tomorrow. Don't pay any attention to the menu, order anything you like — Indonesian, Chinese, Malayan food or, of course, European if you want it. You will hurt his feelings if you just use the menu."

The girls came in; one sat at our table, the other at Hughes'. The effect on the Dutch officers was electrifying.

"Have you ever had a rijstafel?" was the First Mate's opening question to the girl at our table.

"No, but I would love to."

"Good," he said, "We will have lunch tomorrow in my cabin. I'll get the chef to do one of his best."

It appeared that the Engineer also liked rijstafel and the Captain was no slouch either. During the next four days we saw very little of the girls except for an attractive pair of legs mounting the ladder towards the bridge under a notice "Passengers Not Allowed," or a glimpse of a skirt disappearing into a hatch giving access to the engine room. It transpired that the presence of the girls on a more or less twenty-four hour spell of duty was necessary to ensure the safe navigation of the ship and the smooth running of the engines. Sometimes one helped with the navigation and the other with the engines. Sometimes they swapped duties. The Chinese barman did his best to console Hughes and me for the loss of female company.

A ship bound for Shanghai out of Hong Kong joins the established shipping lane, sails through the centre of the Taiwan straits into the China Sea, and is out of sight of land until it reaches the broad estuary of the Yangtze River before turning south into a tributary, the Whang Po. A few miles up the Whang Po stands the city of Shanghai. The captain of our vessel was in no hurry to get there. If necessary he would take his ship himself up the Whang Po but if the pilots' strike was settled — so much the better. He elected to follow the inshore route involving careful navigation from one landfall to another, past a series of lights at night. Constant changes of course, study of charts and alert watch-keeping were demanded.

The route is followed by small coastal craft, junks and fishing vessels; it was much used in the days of sail when weather deteriorated, especially when typhoons threatened. Then a ship would run into a protected anchorage to ride out the storm. As a leisurely exercise the route provides a fascinating spectacle; islands big and small dot the whole length of the coast with the route twisting and turning amongst them. Small villages rest behind beaches. Landlocked coves with their quota of fishing junks, riding at anchor, pass in succession; everywhere are sampans fishing inshore, larger junks trawling nets, huge cargo junks beating up to windward, a dirty coaster or two thrusting against wind and sea to ports such as Swatow and Amoy. The countless islands of the China littoral could be turned entirely or in parts to havens for sun, sea and swimmers — a vast potential holiday archipelago.

As progress is made northwards, the caravel-shaped junks of Southern China give place to the more northern craft with a narrower beam and a painted eye carved on each side of the bow; all have the slatted sails. From these clues an expert can tell the port of origin of a junk by its shape and sail pattern to within a hundred miles along the whole two-thousand mile coast of China.

The bustle of ships ancient and modern increases as the skyline of Shanghai rises from the flat delta country. Built on a mudflat along the Whang Po, some of the buildings lean over crazily as a result of their uneven settlement over the years.

The *Tsidane* tied up right alongside the Bund. Dr Burton was waiting on the wharf, which teemed with coolies, merchants, vendors, officials, customs men, beggars, and rickshaw men.

We got into his car to travel from the Bund through the traffic, swarms of pedestrians, flat carts loaded with merchandise pulled by three coolies, hundreds of bicycle rickshaws, for the four-mile trip to his home on Great Western Road.

"They are well-fed and happy-looking, are they not?" said Burton.

Chapter 4

A MOTLEY GROUP

Fong, Jung et al — A houseboy is sacked — The Compradore and his Cadillac — Model A fords floods — Cold winters and cabotage — Rugby raises my rating — The rise and fall of the CNC.

Doctors Marshall, Jackson and Partners were the only group of British doctors in Shanghai. Tom Burton, one of the Marshall group, was released from internment after World War II together with Paddy Ranson, a member of Jacksons'. During the war, Victor Smolnikoff, a White Russian, had looked after what remained of both practices. Apart from the two interned, only one member, Leo McGolrick, returned. The two groups amalgamated, recruiting George Thorngate, an American, together with a Chinese named Yieh. I was the first new recruit from overseas.

We formed a heterogenous amalgam of nationalities and religions. Tom Burton and I were Scots and Presbyterians. Paddy Ranson was from Northern Ireland, his father a Methodist minister. Leo McGolrick came from Dublin and was a staunch Catholic. George Thorngate from California was a Seventh Day Baptist — very convenient for George as for him Saturday was a religious day, and Sunday was a holiday anyway. Victor Smolnikoff was a Russian Orthodox, and Y. C. Yieh was, as far as we could discover, nothing particular in the religious line. Nationalities and religion were often discussed but I do not remember a diversity of opinion causing any friction.

As in most medical practices in the East, the majority of patients were covered by contracts. The large trading firms were responsible for the medical fees incurred by their foreign staff. This might take the form of the company paying our account, but more generally a blanket sum for all their staff, paid quarterly, covered consultations, hospital visits and so on, but not the cost of surgery or special investigations. Of course, the occasional employee demanded a freedom of choice but the vast majority of British automatically became patients, together with many other nationalities.

We were by far the largest group of doctors in Shanghai, and had two offices, one of which was in the Hong Kong and Shanghai

Bank building on the Bund. The Bund was the famous broad thoroughfare, running along the Whang Po River from the British Consulate grounds of Soochow Creek, past all the main business buildings, to the offices of Taikoo, beyond which a small section formed the river front of the French Concession. All the rest was part of the International Concession. Before the war the concessions enjoyed extraterritorial rights, operating their own police forces, military garrisons, municipal governments and administration. Extraterritorial rights had been surrendered by the Allies at the end of World War II, but the characteristics of the International and French Concessions lived on. The city was run by Mayor Woo. Considering the hotchpotch of nationalities, customs and creeds, he ran it with skill and sagacity; it was no mean task.

From our downtown office on the top floor of the bank we looked over the Bund with its permanent daytime traffic jam of cars, buses, trams, trucks, handcarts, rickshaws and pedicabs — the three-wheel rickshaw with the front a bicycle and the rear a rickshaw type passenger seat. Beyond the thoroughfare were the wharves where junks, sampans and coastal steamers were moored alongside, unloading their cargoes, mostly by coolie labour, onto the waterfront where countless other coolies hefted baskets strung by bamboo poles over their shoulders. Other coolies loaded the cargo into trucks.

From the window, one looked down on a scene of activity which closely resembled a gigantic anthill. Everyone was busy about some business even if it was theft. Right below our office was a section of waterfront reserved for unloading bales of cotton. No one touched the bales until they were loaded onto open trucks, whereupon a group of tough peasant women swarmed forward to grab handfuls of raw cotton and stick the cotton into satchels slung from the waist. Each truck had three coolies with short whips which they wielded, striking at the women. They seldom landed a blow unless one of the women exceeded her quota of about four handfuls. She might then get a nasty lash — deservedly — for breaking the rules. The same women and the same coolies were on duty summer and winter, and no one outside the fraternity got away with anything.

Both our offices, the one on the Bund and the other in the western residential district of Shanghai, had facilities which were comprehensive and at that time in advance of those available in group practices in Europe and many parts of the US. We had our own laboratory and X-ray unit in both offices, with an assortment of secretaries, technicians, nurses and a Chinese "boy" at both. Of these "boys", Fong in the Bank office was nearly fifty and Jung uptown was the oldest employee and very dignified. They both wore long white Chinese gowns.

Fong was a rogue and should have been sacked many times but Burton, who exercised a patriarchal discipline, was loth to "take his rice-bowl from him" as the Chinese expression went. This was a big row when Burton discovered that Fong was conducting his own medical practice in the evenings in our office, dispensing our medicines and drugs — at a net profit for Fong. On another occasion I went into the office in the late evening to find the waiting room crowded. Fong used to let out the space every evening to several families who slept in the warmth and security of the Hong Kong Bank Building, the waiting room being their dormitory. As the elevator boys must have been involved in the racket, the ripples spread to the Bank employees. Fong was caught two mighty blows across his back from Burton's walking stick, a solid instrument, before making good his escape and disappearing for the day. But he was back next day, very contrite in his newly laundered white gown and offering to sacrifice two months' pay for his misdemeanours. "The old bugger," said Smolnikoff, who prided himself on his knowledge of English swear words, "has obviously made at least six months' pay, barring the squeeze given to the watchman and elevator boys!"

Jung, on the other hand, was the epitome of dignity, good manners and decorum. He used to infuriate the senior partners by his sense of propriety. When a patient arrived he would enquire which doctor the patient would want to see. If the patient was a new one, Jung suggested Burton first, then gradually worked down the names till the ultimate ragtag and bobtail was reached, namely me. It did not matter if the others already had several people waiting to see them and I was idle or, as the Chinese would put it, *bak woo ying* — catching flies. To suggest my name first would cause a collective and mounting degree of "loss of face" from Smolnikoff up to Burton. From time to time someone remonstrated with Jung, and very reluctantly and with profound disquiet he would exercise what to a foreigner was common sense — that is, to suggest my name first. A day or two later the proper dignified approach to such matters was resumed.

In the accounts department was the shroff, Mr Chen. The work of a shroff is difficult to define. He received money, totted up cash, paid salaries, was responsible for new Chinese staff, was a mentor and guide to the doctor, interceded with authorites, filled in complicated official forms, and hired people as painters or repairmen, but, most important of all, he knew all the other shroffs, be they shroff of the Shell Company, the National City Bank, the Shanghai Dockyards, the Shanghai Power Company or the Danish East Asiatic Shipping Company. Be the firms big or small, Mr Chen knew them all. Our shroff, who was addressed by everyone as Mr Chen, was about thirty, tall, good-looking, impeccably dressed, usually in a Chinese gown, but sometimes in a finely tailored western suit. Although he considered himself my equal in importance he was invariably polite. He might smile at my ignorance of some custom or official matter, but never gave offence.

One of the houseboy-cooks we had soon after Jean's arrival in Shanghai was surly with Jean, although he gave me good service. One day he demanded an increase in salary. One knew the general standards of pay and our cook was well off, especially as he was on probation. He lost his temper, grabbed my shirt sleeve which tore across and I told him to pack up and go. He then demanded three months' pay before he would leave. There was an impasse. I called up Mr Chen who arrived in no time at all, armed with bundles of notes. As the rate of CNC, that is Chinese National Currency, to the US dollar was 20,000 to one US dollar, and the largest note was a one hundred CNC note, the money was held in bundles of a hundred notes, secured by tape, ten thousand CNC to a bundle. Chen had five or six bundles in the pockets of his gown.

My driver, Chia, and the houseboy sat in the front seat of my car, with Mr Chen and me in the back. We proceeded to the nearest main police station. A large fat policeman stood on a slightly raised platform behind the counter and looked down on us. Chen outlined my complaint and the houseboy then stated his case at great length and very volubly; a few questions were then asked of me. The policeman gazed down at us and delivered his judgement. Six weeks' pay should be given. Mr Chen produced four bundles and placed them on the counter but as the houseboy reached forward in triumph, his hand closing on the first bundle, the huge hand of the policeman came down hard on top. Nobody moved for several seconds till the policeman slowly lifted the houseboy's arm and moved it back from the counter. The policeman then took three bundles and put them on a table behind him. His stern glance embraced us all. He handed one bundle to the houseboy and said to him, "If you are not out of the house in half an hour you will be arrested."

Mr Chen came back to our flat to make sure that the houseboy left with only his belongings and not ours. While having a cup of tea I complained of the costs of the rough and ready justice meted out by the police constable.

"Dr Wedderburn," said Chen, "we did very well, I think." He put his hands into the deep pockets of his gown to take out several more bundles of money.

"I brought along three months' pay, just in case," he said.

The position of shroff in large companies gradually merged into that of a compradore, or head middle-man, who conducted trading negotiations on behalf of his employers. A good shroff-compradore could become a very rich man. The compradore of the Shell Oil Company of China worked in the Shell Company building on the Bund. Because of his prestige and position he used the imposing front entrance. For him to emerge at five o'clock to climb into his huge Cadillac, possibly at the same time as the Managing Director's smaller car drew up, would cause the Manager to lose face. Promptly at five a magnificent blue and gold rickshaw pulled by two men in matching uniforms halted in front of the Shell building. The compradore emerged, sat back on the luxurious seat and was pulled at a sharp trot up the side road to the back of the building. If he passed one of the European employees he would bow and raise his hand in salutation. In the back street he dismounted to step into his waiting Cadillac. From that moment on no one would expect to be shown any sign of recognition. This was right and proper conduct.

The firm had to provide me with a car, which was not an easy commodity to come by, but an old Model A Ford, the successor of the Model T, became my property. The great thing about a Model A was that the engine and works were so basic and simple that nothing ever went wrong with them. By dint of cracking through the gears, a fair turn of acceleration and speed could be achieved. True, it was not the smooth limousine of a successful surgeon, but it served me well. However, the fact that it stood so high on its wheels was a disadvantage. Shanghai was built on a mudflat only a few feet above sea-level, and when heavy rain fell the streets became flooded. My Model A was the only car in the practice which could negotiate the floods so I used to find myself doing seven people's work until the waters subsided.

My driver Chia was invariably willing and cheerful. When Jean arrived in Shanghai in May, her steamer tied up at a wharf on the Bund. Immediately vast mobs of coolies, customs men, agents, peddlers, thieves and money changers poured on board. Chia and I jostled our way up the gangway to greet Jean and our daughter Corinna, then seventeen months old. While Jean and I fussed with baggage and documents, Chia lifted Corinna in his arms to set off with her to the Model A. Jean looked around for Corinna, and glanced over onto the wharf to see a strange Chinese disappearing with our daughter.

"Someone has kidnapped Corinna!" she said with wild alarm, thinking that this had happened even before she had set foot on China's soil.

"Don't worry, dear, he is my driver," I replied. But Jean was on tenterhooks till we got to the car to find Corinna sitting on Chia's lap and happily sounding the horn, a sound barely audible over the roar of vehicles and humanity.

Chia stayed with us throughout our time in Shanghai. After we left he escaped to Hong Kong. There we tried to get him a job but he failed his driving test. He had had no experience of starting on a hill, as every road in Shanghai was dead flat; the only incline in the whole city was the approach to the bridge over Soochow Creek. He did succeed later in passing the test, and got a job as driver for Douglas Clague, who rose to head one of the largest trading companies. He became Sir Douglas Clague, and every now and then I see Chia standing beside the Lincoln Continental or the Rolls Royce waiting for Sir Douglas. Despite his elevation to the cars of the mighty, Chia still gives me the same old grin and when Corinna or Alexi, who was born in Shanghai, are out in Hong Kong, Chia will appear to greet them and hand them a present.

Until Jean arrived I stayed with Burton and McGolrick in Burton's house on Great Western Road. The Shanghai winters are cold, and ice forms on the streets in the late afternoon. Heating was a big problem and many diverse forms of heating were in use. At Burton's there was an iron stove in the lounge from which a pipe started upwards and then sagged sideways through a couple of insecure bends to discharge through a hole in the wall.

Coal was £100 a ton, a lot of money in those days, as China invoked the law of cabotage and forbade foreign ships to carry coal or any cargo between Chinese ports. In theory this was fine, but in practice China had no ships. Before the war, coal had been carried from Chingwantao near the Kailan mines to Shanghai by the Kailan mine company's own colliers. The mines were operated by a foreign consortium which would not, because of cabotage, build or hire ships, so the coal supplies were erratic in their arrival and extremely expensive. The foolish chauvinistic application of the cabotage laws meant that much commercial cargo, carried along the coast by the famous Yangtze river steamers, ceased to move at all. The Chinese had neither the ships nor the know-how to operate the coastal and river trade. This resulted in the stifling of trade and was just one more factor adding to the difficulties and hopelessness of the Nationalist cause. The coastal trade was of vital importance because the railways between the Yangtze valley and the north were permanently cut by the Communists.

It was not much fun living with two senior partners. Although Burton by all accounts had been a real rip in his younger days, he frowned on any social activities of mine, especially those that kept me out late. As the security arrangements at night were stringent, a late return in the early hours meant waking the houseboy, who slept soundly, to be followed by a loud drawing of bolts, keys turning rusty locks and a general hullabaloo calculated to wake the neighbourhood.

Burton's houseboy had started years before when a lad as the keeper of Burton's dogs, succeeding his ancient father as houseboy. The father still lived in the kitchen and servants' quarters. No matter at what time of the day one entered the kitchen, the father had a pair of shoes in his hands; these he was polishing assiduously. This activity, the excuse for his presence, developed as a result of Burton entering the kitchen on one of Shanghai's hot, humid August evenings to find the old man stretched out on a camp bed, the refrigerator door open and the old man's feet resting on the bottom shelf. He made his exit as Burton advanced, wielding his walking stick. We never found out nor dared ask whether Burton's ire was raised principally on account of the possible contamination of the food or the thought of the increased electricity bill.

I managed quite inadvertently to raise my prestige with Burton, by joining the Shanghai Rugby Club. Because of the restraint on my social activities I was soon physically fitter than many of the other members, working my way into the first fifteen and playing for Shanghai in the annual big match, the Interport against Hong Kong.

As Burton had played for Glasgow Academicals before he lost

his leg in World War I, when according to him they had won the Scottish Championship, I went up in his estimation. During the Interport, the hardest and toughest game I ever played, the score was three all with five minutes to go, when I picked up the ball in a loose scrimmage and scored the winning try.

Burton was delighted, grudgingly giving me the only words of praise he ever bestowed on me: "You played not a bad game."

The next year I was captain, but our membership shrank as the Communist forces approached. We were a hopeful but unbalanced team when we flew to Hong Kong for the last Interport and suffered a resounding defeat. Later, the very last rugby match in China was played against a team from the cruiser HMS *London* in April 1949. On winding-up, the committee found that the club was well off financially and it was suggested that on dissolution we approach the English Rugby Union and furnish a Shanghai room at Twickenham, the home of English rugby, as a memorial to the long history of the Shanghai Rugby Club. This scheme did not get off the ground as the treasurer disappeared to Australia with the proceeds of the club and a good deal more of his firm's money. It was some consolation to hear many months afterwards that he had continued to exercise his talents in Australia, and was languishing in gaol with a year's sentence for embezzlement.

In the year of my arrival, 1947, Shanghai was booming, and the future looked buoyant. China under Chiang Kai-shek was at last free and able to forge ahead from the chaos of a war which had started in 1937 with the Japanese contrived "incident" at the Marco Polo bridge near Peking. American aid of all descriptions poured in. To make up for years of deprivation, goods cascaded onto every dock in Shanghai and everyone had a finger in the pie. Certainly there were warning signals: a rip-roaring inflation, graft of national proportion, rampant corruption, and wheeling and dealing of every kind. But it was possible, in fact probable, that freedom and unity could be achieved, malpractices brought under restraint and a prosperous country created. That the common sense, frugality and the infinite capacity for hard work of the Chinese would result in a new China better run than ever before was not a foolish hope.

Apart from the misfortunes of the German mark after the First World War, there can never have been such a steady, relentless depreciation of a currency as that which befell CNC, the Chinese National Currency. The first question you asked a friend at lunch time was, "What is the rate?"

I used to get a fair idea of the rate by buying a packet of Chesterfield cigarettes from the woman outside the entrance to our office in the Bank building. It might be CNC 20,000 in the morning and 22,000 by evening. One's interest was far from academic; unconsciously one knew if goods were expensive or cheap without having to do a mental calculation converting to US dollars. Everyone soon developed this sixth sense, and problems differed from person to person. I drew my cash from our office at the rate of the day, being debited against a basic pay in Hong Kong dollars, but people who were paid in CNC once a month might find the money depreciated to a third by the end of the month. They had to change the money into US dollars, silver dollars or ounces of gold, and change it back into small amounts for their daily needs. One or two foreign firms allowed their staff to draw money at the prevailing rate at the beginning of the month and pay it back at the exchange rate of the last day of the month. Most of their groceries were bought early in the month to be paid back at a third of their value. Needless to say the staff of these firms were the envy of all other mortals.

In August 1948, CNC was abolished and a new currency, Gold Yuan, introduced at four to the US dollar. By dint of the threat of the death penalty for dealing in currency, and one or two unfortunates were executed, the exchange rate held for almost two months. Victor Smolnikoff, impressed by the arrest of some people and more so by the death penalty, suddenly blossomed forth in a succession of new suits; as he had not been sartorially conscious previously, I asked him what the change was all about.

"Well I have to turn the money into something, don't I?" he replied.

Some nine months later the receipt for our monthly milk bill was forty-two million Gold Yuan.

Chia, my driver, was paid weekly. He immediately purchased crates of bottled orange juice. Though in fact he did not take physical possession of the crates; it was a credit transaction with the local shop. He would then sell back a crate or two from day to day at the new rate to cover his daily purchases. Everyone had his own method.

Internal airline pilots were the best off as the rate nearly always slipped faster in Shanghai than in, for instance, Hankow. A pilot could buy one million CNC in Shanghai for US$100. Arriving in Handow the same day he could sell the million for US$110 — he was making money coming and going! Every now and then the rate might go the other way and the airline pilots with their suitcases of currency would actually lose on the deal. Their indignation was expressed loudly, and greeted raucously by everyone else with the comment, "Our hearts bleed for you, buddy!"

Every evening a dealer called at our office and took the spare cash, giving a credit slip against Hong Kong dollars. Chen, the shroff, told me the dealer distributed this cash next morning to his clientele of Chinese who were receiving foreign currency remittances from relatives abroad.

Before my arrival in Shanghai, the Royal Navy had given China a cruiser and a destroyer to bolster her navy. The Admiralty in London insisted on having the crews sent to Britain for training and on having them medically examined. Only McGolrick, Thorngate and Smolnikoff were in Shanghai and although the complement for training was about fifteen hundred men, by the time that number were found fit, over three thousand men had been examined. The examinations, including chest X-rays and blood and urine samples, took place in the hot, humid summer evenings after normal office hours and was no mean task for three doctors. The bill was the equivalent in CNC of approximately US$8,000, but Doctors Marshall, Jackson and Partners could hardly adopt the procedure of quoting it in US dollars, and had to quote it in CNC. By the time the Chinese Government paid the bill some eight months later, it was equivalent to nine or ten US dollars. Although Smolnikoff's arithmetic was always suspect, his statement may have been correct when he said that in the end they had examined each candidate for "one-third of one damn bloody US cent!"

Chapter 5

THE SOVIET CITIZEN AND OTHERS

Film shows at the consulate — An unusual baptism — Natasha and anaesthesia — Obtaining a medical licence — Bryant's brassy cough.

Victor Smolnikoff and I got on well together right from the start. We were both in our early thirties, separated from Yieh and Thorngate by ten years, and by more than twenty from the seniors.

In China there must have been a few hundred thousand Russians who had escaped during the revolution. Victor's parents had been working on the stretch of railway from Harbin to the Russian border, where it became the Trans-Siberian Railway. They were in Manchuria during the revolution and never went back. Most of the White Russians were a feckless lot, reliving the past in Russia and hopelessly ineffectual in facing their present and future in China. The fact that the Smolnikoffs had given their son a good education and put him through medicine in Shanghai was exceptional. He did not have Slavonic features; a stranger might have taken him for an Anglo-Saxon. His English was faultless and without an accent, but he was not truly bilingual because there were many words he did not know as he had neither heard them nor read them.

Shortly after my arrival he was sent off to Scotland for postgraduate training, ostensibly in dermatology, but under the wing of Sir James Learmonth he was side-tracked and he developed an interest in anaesthesia which ultimately was of supreme importance to him. He was very popular in Edinburgh, being something of a seven-day wonder — a novelty who nevertheless kept people amused because of his critical but gentle sense of humour onto which were grafted his stories and experiences.

As the Communists grew more powerful, the Russians looked for avenues of escape. They had neither passports nor official nationality; they had to be accepted as immigrants to other countries. Lack of education, basic skills and training did not endear them to countries which exercised a discriminatory immigration policy. But Smolnikoff was among a select few, educated, with a record of service to his fellowmen during the war years. Both the Canadian and Australian consuls told him that both he and his family would be welcomed.

NO LOTUS GARDEN

His wife was a staunch Russian. Unlike Victor she spoke only Russian, and did not encourage the children, six in number, to speak anything but Russian at home. After much soul-searching Victor decided to apply for Soviet papers. All of us in the firm were dismayed and saddened but had no alternative to accepting his conclusion.

When at last they all had passports, Victor was invited to a film show and drinks at the Russian Consulate, the signal of success.

"How did it go?" I enquired the next day.

"Well," said Smolnikoff, "it was a bit of a mixed blessing. First we had some drinks."

"Vodka or what?" I asked.

"Scotch whisky, of course. Then we saw the film, a bunch of workers in a steel factory; it only lasted fifteen minutes which was quite enough. Then the Consul got up to make a speech about all the poor Russians in Shanghai, suggesting that we made a contribution."

"Mr Udal," said the Consul to a very successful furrier, "I suggest that you should start the ball rolling."

Comrade Udal heaved himself to his feet, and took a deep breath before offering a cheque for US$500.

The Consul glanced at the paper in his hand.

"Comrade Udal," he said, "I have you down for three thousand dollars."

Smolnikoff's heart sank as the Consul worked down the list. Victor was at the very bottom. When his turn came he offered two hundred and fifty. The Consul glanced over his glasses at Victor.

"Thank you, Doctor Smolnikoff," he said.

"Heck," remarked Victor to me, "I was ready to talk about being a very junior partner, having six children with my wife pregnant. I considered offering up to five hundred or down to fifty. Obviously I hit the nail right on the bloody head."

"Serves you right, Comrade S," I said.

Some two months afterwards Smolnikoff was sitting rivetted into his office chair, holding a printed card at which he gazed.

"What's that?" I asked.

"Another invitation to a film show at the Consulate."

Next morning I said, "How much, Victor?"

"Oh, much better, only fifty dollars."

One of the major troubles of having a Russian, White or Red, as an employer and friend was the manner in which one was entertained. Where alcohol is concerned, Russians have no discrimination or method, except possibly to follow a policy of total catholicism.

When his seventh child was delivered, Jean and I attended the christening in their apartment. Immediately on entering, a glass of something potent was thrust into our hands; the ceremony soon got under way with an Orthodox priest conducting affairs. The priest lifted the baby. In the centre of the lounge was a large tin bath. The priest started to chant while walking in circles round the bath, followed by the guests in line; each guest clutched a glass from which he refreshed himself. The line stopped moving occasionally as we drank a toast before getting on the way again. Everyone joined in this slow march except two minions who stationed themselves strategically on the periphery. Their duty was to replenish our glasses while we were on the move in case we ran out of fuel. It did not matter what was in the glass — possibly it might be half full of vermouth when a large dollop of crème de menthe would be added first time around, maybe rum on the next circuit; anything handy!

Finally the baby was dunked in the bath, not a quick in and out but a good solid immersion. Possibly the priest's appreciation of the time a baby could be held under water without being drowned was prejudiced by the alcohol concentration in the blood supplying his brain cells.

The select assembled company then proceeded to celebrate, but whether this was on account of the christening or the baby's survival was not immediately clear. The festivities wound up with dinner. Not content with filling our glasses, from time to time Victor's arm would reach over our shoulders to pour from unidentifiable bottles a liberal measure into the soup bowl or over the meat and vegetables. This is the only Russian Orthodox christening Jean and I have attended. One was quite enough. Perhaps it was the finale for the Smolnikoffs, because after the seventh child the production line ground to a halt.

Smolnikoff had established himself as our anaesthetist. The only gas available in Shanghai was oxygen but he had returned from his trip abroad with a Mackintosh vaporiser. This machine, soon superseded in Europe, was an effective device and stood us in good stead. The principle of the machine was to vaporise ether, the vapour being delivered to what would now be considered a clumsy mask. The use of the mask interfered with the surgeon's operating field if he was working on a patient's neck.

It gradually dawned on us a few months later that Smolnikoff had succumbed to a grand passion, becoming deeply involved with Natasha, a recent graduate from the same medical school. As the approach of the Communists was causing a contraction of legitimate business activity, it was not easy for a girl to get started in practice and Smolnikoff was able to further his courtship under the guise of teaching Natasha the basis of anaesthesia. The two of them officiated at the top of the table while I was working at mid-level. It was Burton who, while assisting me, had time to register what was going on. With characteristic paternal emphasis he reproved Smolnikoff when we were drinking tea after the operation.

"Look here, Smolnikoff," he remarked, "I don't approve, but if you must further your sexual relations, I would be obliged if you would conduct your affairs outside the operating theatre."

Thereafter Natasha only appeared when someone else's case was under treatment, but little progress was being made about finding her qualified employment.

Natasha was quite a good looking girl and as I was the recipient of a blow-by-blow account of progress towards a job and other more personal matters, my interest was inevitably aroused so that I also was concerned when Dr Bernikoff entered the arena. Bernikoff seemed to me to enjoy some fundamental advantages in his relations with Natasha, being not only unmarried and in his twenties, but also unburdened by seven children. Bernikoff worked in the medical analysis laboratory, a private laboratory run by a Dr Lempert.

Lempert was also a White Russian who had great energy and drive. He possessed an immense degree of charm and always appeared as though his suit had come straight from Savile Row. In the face of difficulties which would have deterred a lesser man, he ran a superb laboratory and organised Shanghai's first blood bank. Lempert was settled in Shanghai but would have to leave before the Communists arrived, because as a youth he had escaped from Vladivostok to Korea and was very much a "wanted man" by the Russians. When the time came for him to depart he would hand the laboratory over to Bundikoff, the elderly radiologist who ran the X-ray side of the business.

Bernikoff and Smolnikoff first approached Bundikoff regarding a job for Natasha, but he, although heir apparent, had to have Lempert's agreement. The day came when Victor took Natasha to see Lempert. I was agog to hear the result when Victor burst into my

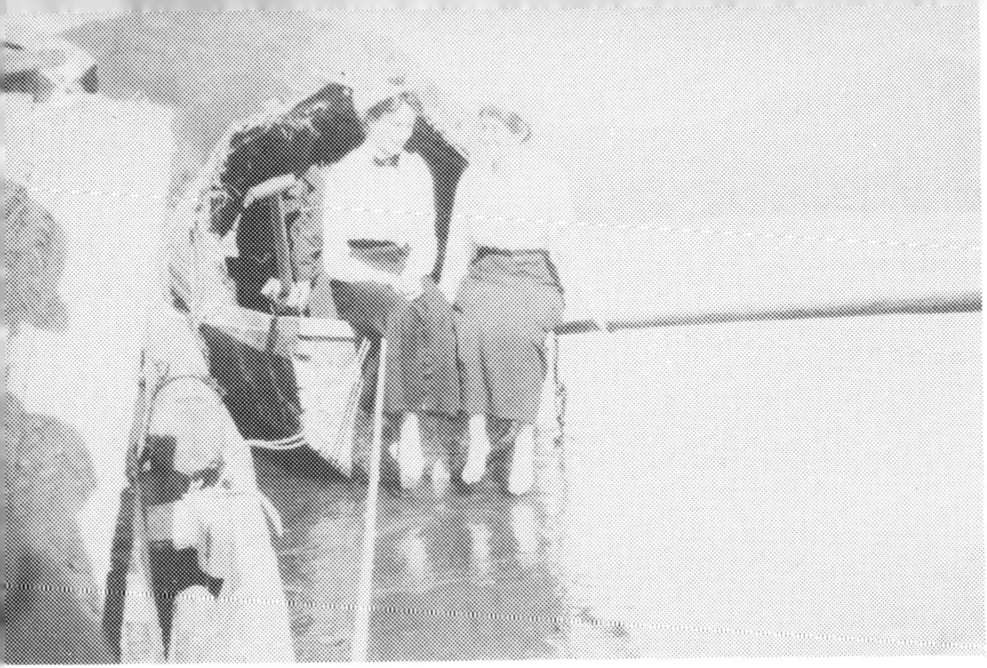

My mother (right) *and friend on the Sungari on the way to Kirin.*

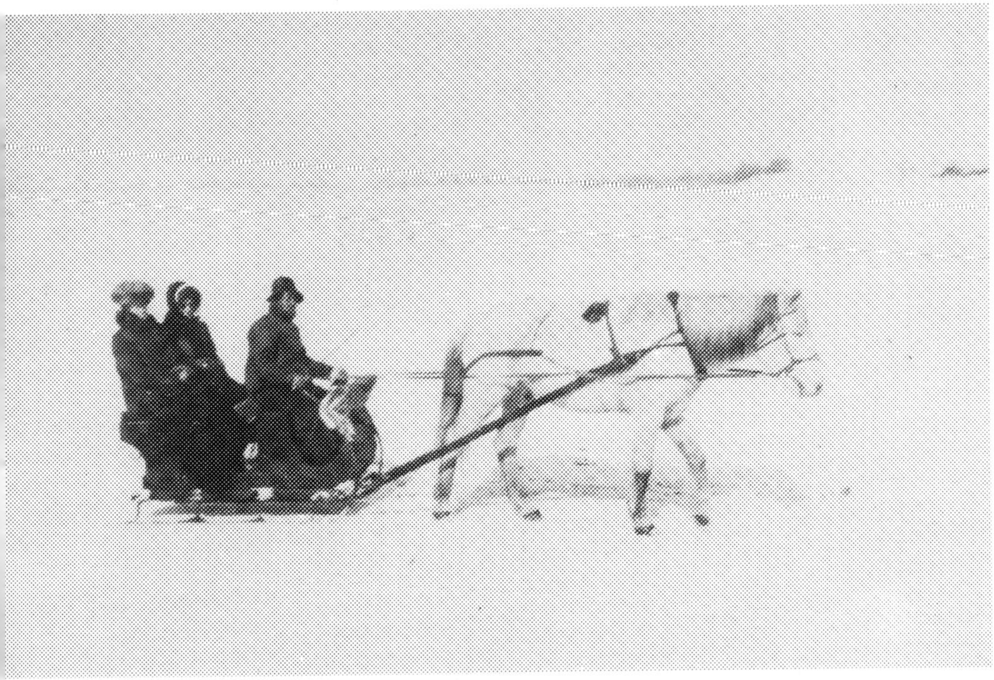

On the frozen Sungari.

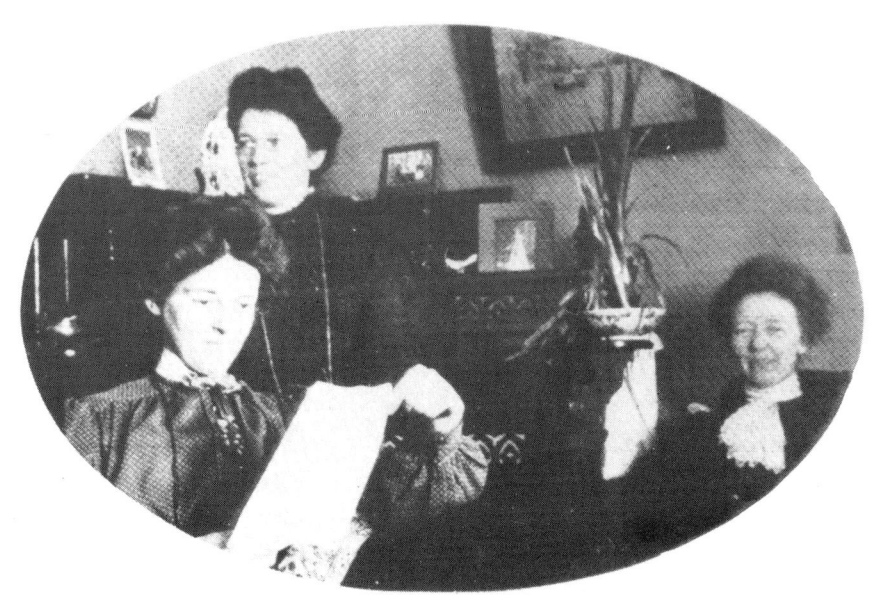

At home in Kirin.

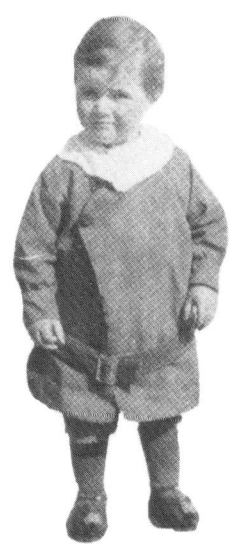

(Left) *The author aged one year.*

(Below) *Aunt Emma* (left) *and our family at Kirin in 1917.*

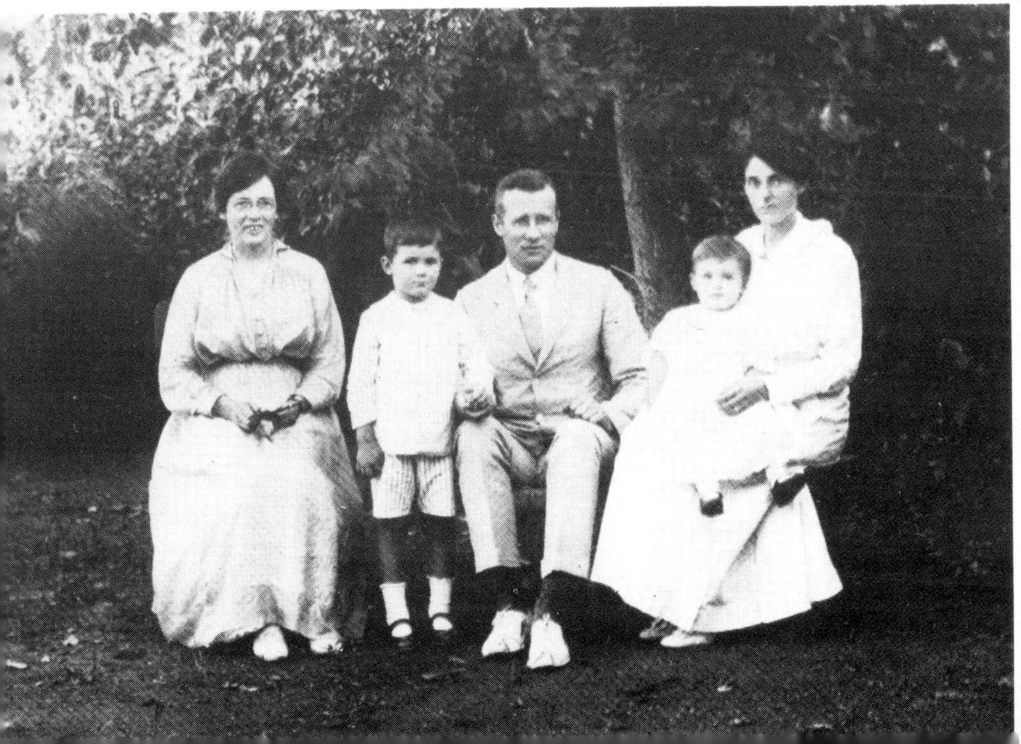

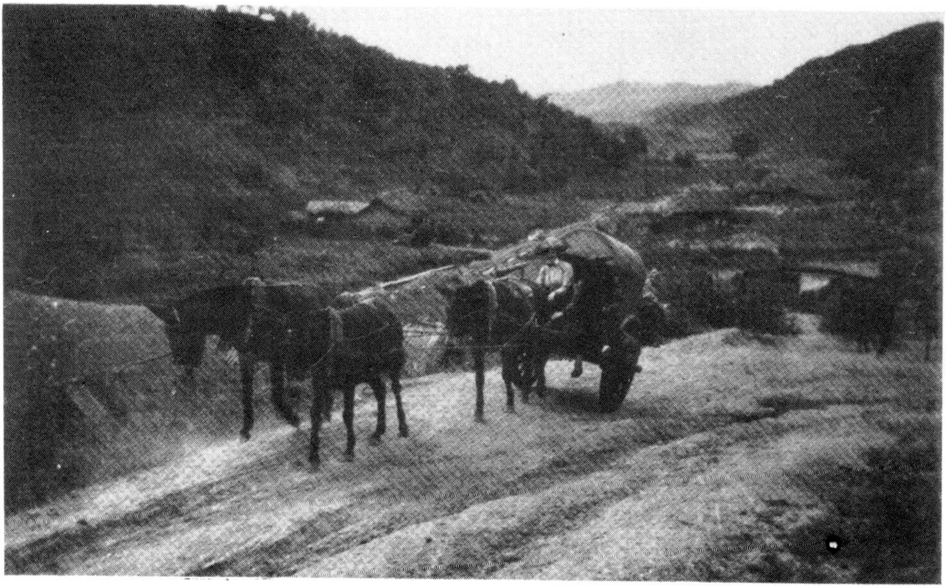

My mother returning home from Mukden in 1912.

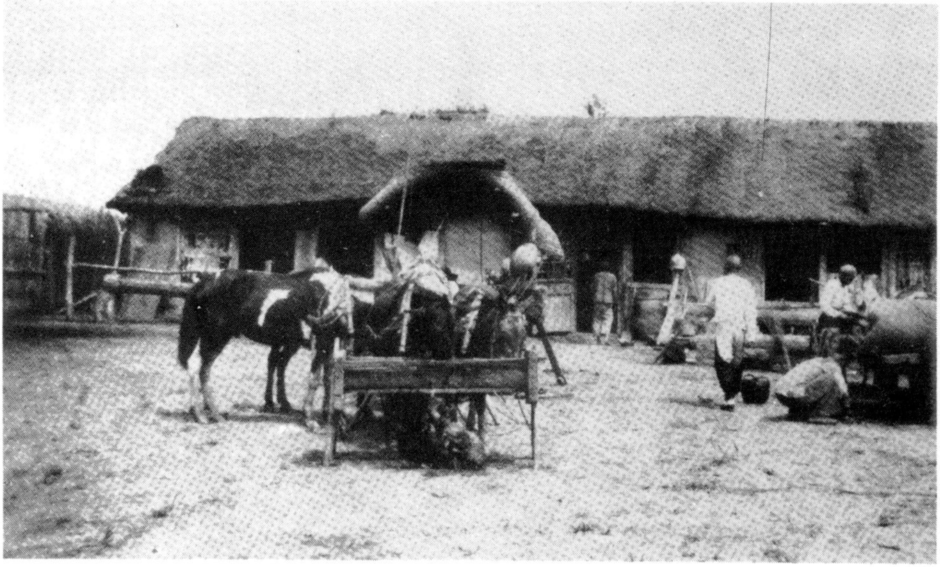

Scene outside a small Chinese inn.

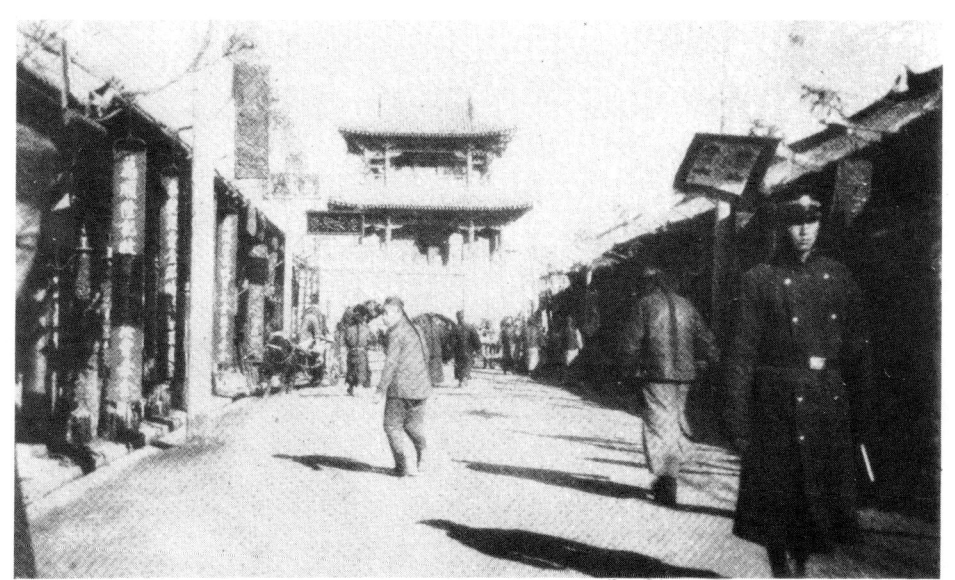

Street in Mukden.

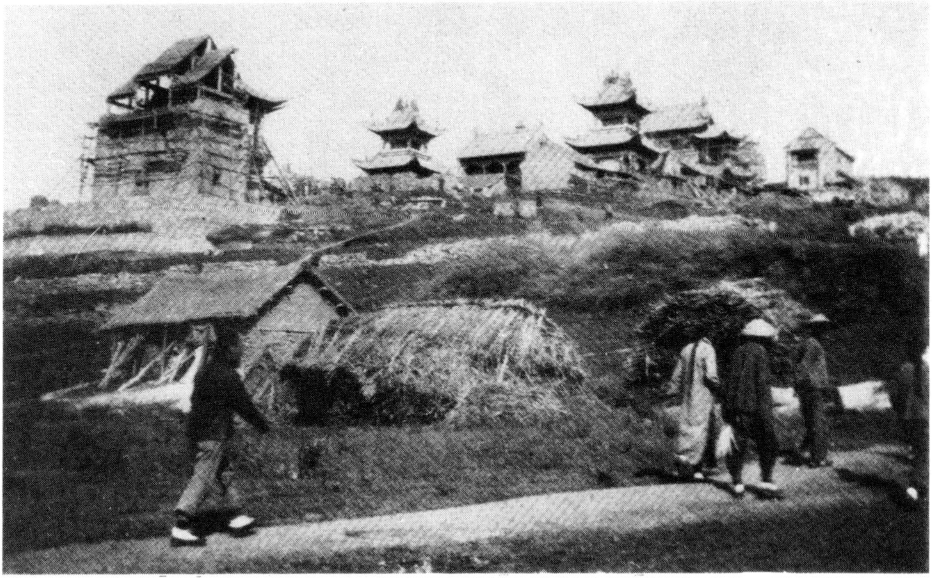

Temple construction in progress near Kirin.

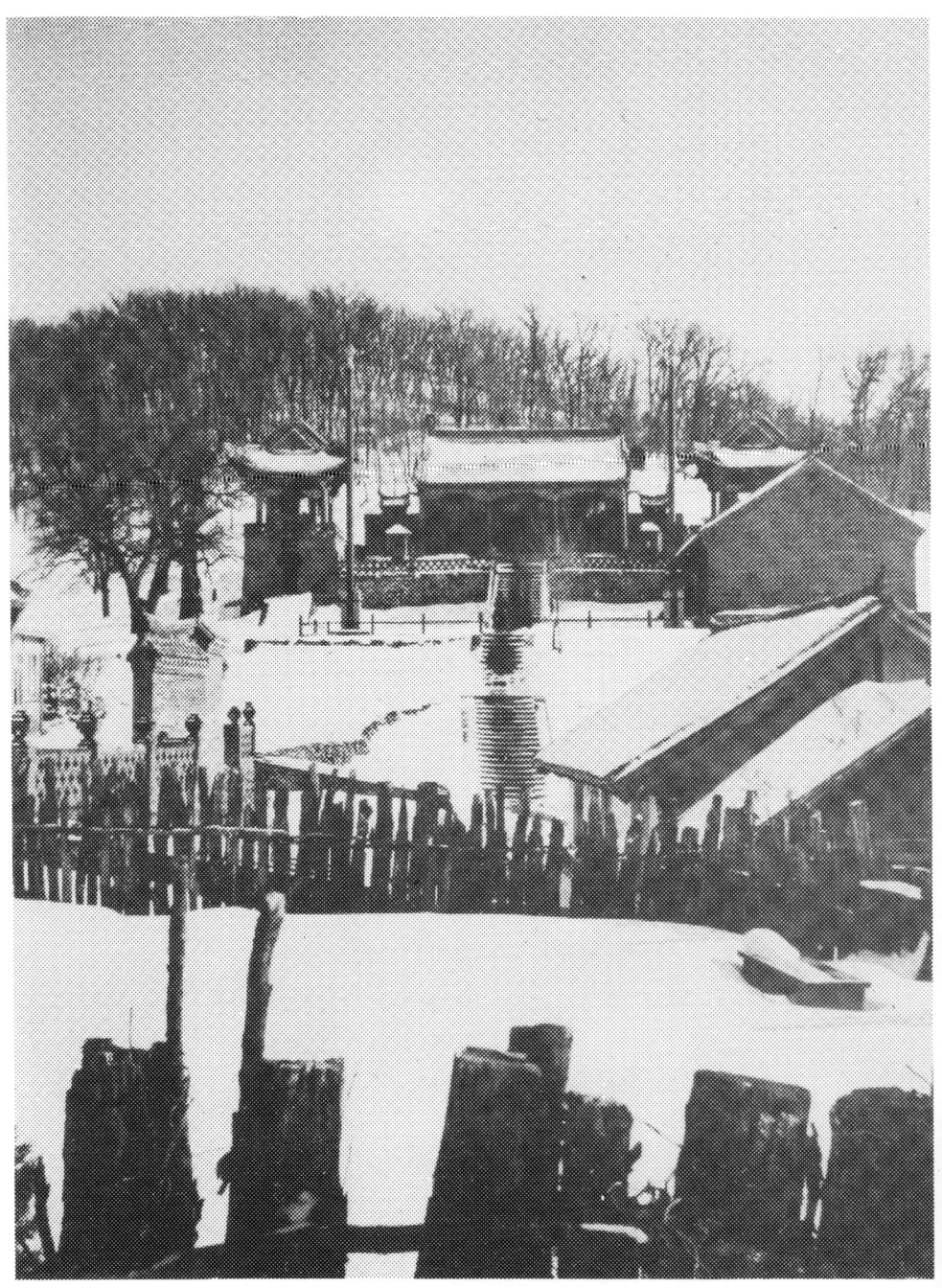

Temple at the top of Lung Tan Shan, Kirin.

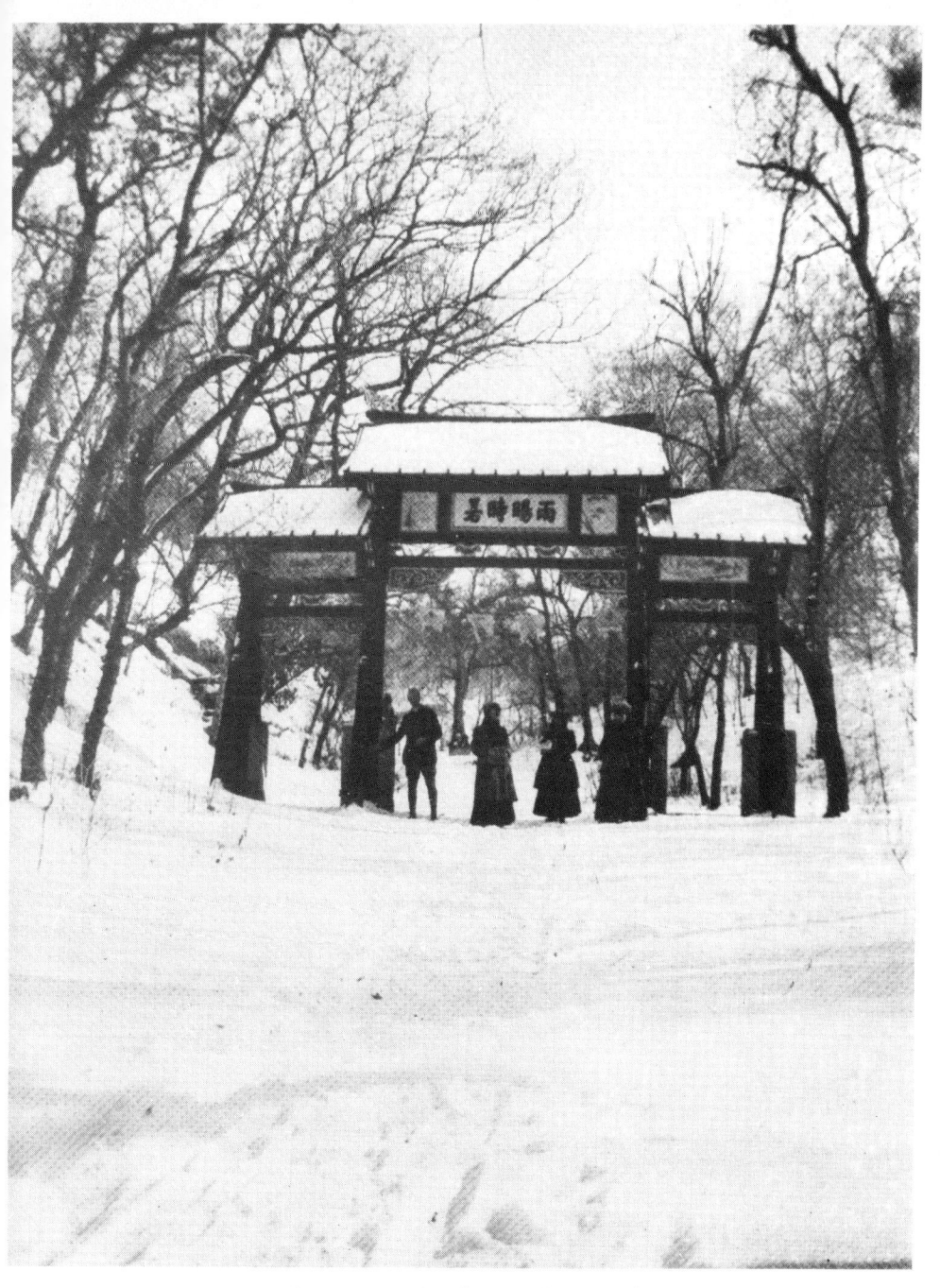

The gateway leading to the temple.

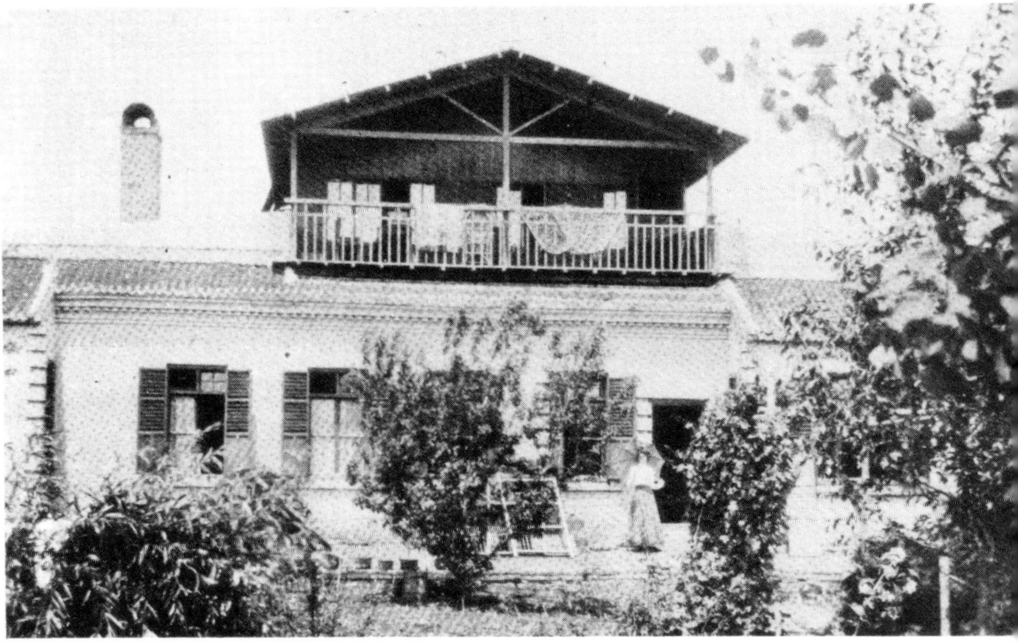

The house at Chao Yang Chun.

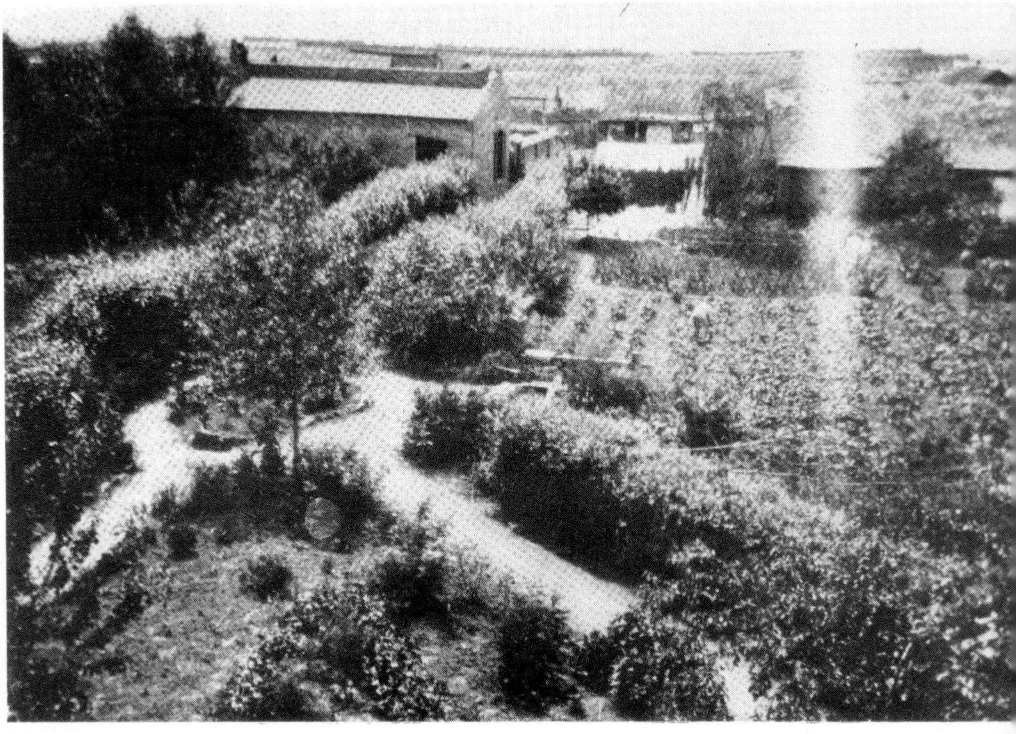

The garden.

office to tell me that all was well, and would I join Natasha and him and Bernikoff and Bundikoff at the Russian Sporting Club that evening.

Smolnikoff and I were there first. We sat on the lawn. He pointed out to me some parallel bars in a corner across the grass.

"Do you know, Gren," he said, "we Russians are absolutely hopeless. I am the convener of the sports committee; if we moved the parallel bars to that other corner we would enlarge the football pitch, but although we passed it a year ago it has been top subject on the general committee agenda in countless meetings. Someone, not always the same person, objects, so that this simple thing is still stalled after hours of discussion. We Russians cannot agree on even the simplest resolution. We talk, argue, swallow vodka, and postpone the decision from sheer exhaustion. That is why we must have a man like Stalin.

"Stalin tells us what to do and we had better do it or we are up against a wall looking down the wrong end of rifle barrels. I tell you, Gren, although you consider him a monster, a man like Stalin is absolutely essential for Russia."

Bernikoff arrived as this homily ended. All was bonhomie and geniality; Bundikoff joined us so that congratulations were exchanged all round. No one worried about Natasha until she was over an hour late; concern was not really manifest for another half hour. Smolnikoff telephoned her home. She had gone out dressed for an occasion. We all sat baffled, fortifying ourselves with vodka, till a horrible thought crossed Bernikoff's mind. Had the smooth-working Lempert decided to entertain Natasha himself?

There were more phone calls; Lempert was not in the French Club, his evening home from home. The telephone in his flat went unanswered. We helped Bernikoff start his motor bike into action before he sped off. Meanwhile, Bundikoff, puffing at his pipe, advanced the idea that our worst fears were probably justified. Bernikoff returned, he had stopped opposite Lempert's home in Cathay Mansions. Yes the lights were on in Lempert's sixth floor apartment but no one answered the door bell. The trouble was we could not be absolutely sure. It was an occasion which suited the Russian temperament. The rivals were now allies in adversity, and I half expected them to break into some emotional song. Round midnight I refused Bernikoff's offer of a lift on the back of his motorcycle; we took a taxi, dropping Victor off to the bosom of his family.

As I got out of the taxi, Bundikoff said to me, "And that, I think, is that."

Yieh was a very different person from Smolnikoff. He was a demon for work. If I called him up to ask him to help me with a case he would say, "OK. I am coming."

"Oh Yieh," I would quickly have to shout down the phone, "not now, tomorrow morning at nine," or he would have been on his way.

Yieh and I took a trip to Nanking in order to get my medical licence. Nanking had suffered greatly during the war. There were few private cars but hosts of army trucks and jeeps which hurtled down sodden streets, crashing through pools of water, sending showers of muddy water on pedestrians. It was bitterly cold, and it rained for all four days without ceasing. We checked in to a Chinese hotel to find there was only one room free, which had a large double bed, so we shared it. At night Yieh got down to his longjohns, garments which I wished I 'had had. We had Chinese food for breakfast, lunch and dinner; no one likes Chinese food better than I do, but a Western stomach needs an alternative.

In the mornings we visited the Foreign Office and the Ministry of Health, waiting in various draughty offices for hours. In the afternoons we went sightseeing, sometimes in a jeep, sometimes on foot. We lumbered along Nanking's wall in the rain, climbed the seven hundred steps to Sun Yat Sen's tomb in the rain, scaled pagodas in the rain. One afternoon we visited a hot springs bath house, a relic of the Japanese occupation. It was a soldiers' convalescent home with a huge bath of steaming-hot water in which half a battalion of Chinese soldiers was immersed. The commandant offered us a bath which I accepted before Yieh could demur; it seemed to me to be the only chance of getting warm.

"With all these soldiers I hope we don't get VD," said Yieh.

As I gently lowered myself into the scalding water I told him, "No self-respecting gonococcus or spirochaete could remain alive in this for more than five seconds."

On our last afternoon, tramping along some dingy side street, Yieh asked me if I would like some afternoon tea. A vision of buttered toast, scones and jam floated in front of me. "Yes, good idea," I instantly replied. Yieh immediately dodged up a dark stairway to a crowded tea house and placed the order. Up came a huge plateful of dark and greasy noodles.

Soon afterwards we boarded the night train to Shanghai and

were hardly settled in the double first-class sleeping car when the attendant asked me if I would like toast, bacon and eggs. I was grasped by an intense elation but summoned all my resolve to refuse. Yieh would have thought it impolite for me to start right away on uncivilised Western food so soon after the sumptuous "afternoon tea". The licence arrived a few days later, a magnificent document on red paper emblazoned at the top with the Nationalist flag.

Yieh, Smolnikoff and I were all involved in the odd case of Bryant, the Lutheran missionary. For some reason best known to themselves, this group had a mission in the Lola country in the far west of China; a wild and mountainous region close to Tibet. The mission had a DC-3 aircraft to fly in supplies and staff. The Lola were best described as aborigines, and flying at least assured arrival. For missionaries to trek in would result in a few unmarked graves.

Bryant had developed a very peculiar complaint. If he bent his head backwards he developed a terrible fit of coughing which lasted for two or three minutes. He was careful to avoid making this movement, but in the pulpit his enthusiasm to proclaim the Word of the Lord would sooner or later cause him to raise his eyes toward heaven and throw his head back, so that the sermon and service were brought to a sudden stop.

In medical textbooks, certain signs have special labels; one such is a cough described as a "brassy cough". When Bryant put back his head to stimulate the onset of a coughing fit, one immediately realised that one was hearing for the first time a brassy cough. There simply is no other way of describing the noise that came forth; the description brassy is perfect. I have never heard such a cough again.

He was seen by various doctors. The reason for his complaint could not be ascertained, but an old American doctor who had been a professor of Ear, Nose and Throat, remembered that the external laryngeal nerve had been divided in the past to relieve the pain of the larynx in intractable cases of tuberculosis. The professor and others concluded that the lateral external laryngeal nerve should be divided; they persuaded me to do this. If this was not successful, no doubt I would bear the blame. One difficulty was that Smolnikoff's anaesthetic mask would get in the way, so it was decided to block the upper neck nerves with local anaesthesia as they emerged from the spine. I followed the instructions in a textbook to the letter, but some local anaesthetic got into the spinal canal, effectively paralysing all the muscles of respiration. Fortunately this responded to artificial respiration and passed off in a few minutes. It is an uncommon procedure to expose the membrane of the larynx, which turned out to be gossamer thin, bulging in and out with every breath; the nerve was a mere filament. I put a little local round it. Bryant's head was then extended back over the end of the operating table, but he did not cough. "Praise be to the Lord!" he said. My advisers had made a correct diagnosis and chosen the correct nerve, the left not the right. I divided the nerve.

Bryant spent the next day sitting up, and bending his head back. When discharged from hospital he paid his bill at the office, walked through the front door, threw back his head to sing a hymn of rejoicing and fell down the steps! He was promptly re-admitted. Three days later Smolnikoff gave him an aeaesthetic, and I assisted Yieh when he exposed the medial cartilage of Bryant's right knee to find the cartilage completely torn across.

You can't keep a good man down; he was off back to the Lola country in a couple of weeks, climbing the mountains, exhorting his flock, raising his arms to greet his God, and holding his head back to gaze up at the sky.

Chapter 6

AN ESCAPE

A meeting with Robert Lim — O.P. escapes — Sino-Scottish relationships.

The world press was so weary of the Chinese war that it warranted hardly a paragraph, much less headlines. Thus an epic battle took place and went unnoticed. The greatest engagement ever fought on Chinese soil and one of the decisive major battles of our own or any previous age took place virtually unreported.

Where the Peking-Tientsin to Nanking railway is bisected by the lateral Lang Hui railway is the town of Tsuchow, the gateway from North to Central China. Over this ground the Communist and the Nationalist armies, numbering nearly three quarters of a million men on each side, slugged it out from late November 1948 to January 1949. The Nationalists, routed, fell back to behind the line of the Yangtze, arranged a three month armistice, and tried to negotiate a division of China — all to the north to be Communist and all to the south to remain with the Nationalists, or Kuomintang, under the suzerainty of Chiang Kai-shek. Tsuchow town itself held out for another month before its garrison surrendered.

The Communists knew that no effective army remained, and rejected any compromise.

In Shanghai we were only dimly aware of the magnitude of the disaster until wounded soldiers started to appear on the streets. Armies in China from time immemorial had been feared. The common soldier was the scum of the earth, greedy and rapacious in victory, transformed into a ruthless brigand by defeat. The wounded men, suffering and hungry, did not excite sympathy nor receive help. The Chinese population exhibited that typical characteristic with which they can greet unpleasantness. They totally ignored it, but it was no good pretending that the soldiers were not there. There were too many for that.

For reasons which were never explained, a few soldiers found their way into a hospital in which I did a round once a week. A soldier might be on a bed or even the floor, his wounded limb wrapped in newspaper; no chart hung from the bed or the wall. If they received treatment, there was no evidence of it. Once or twice I stopped to try to examine one soldier but this caused embarrassment. Week after week the same men lay there, obviously ill, abandoned, their lack-lustre eyes showing only a momentary flicker of interest before their spirits again withdrew into a shroud of suffering. As many were peasant boys from faraway provinces speaking only their local dialects, the language barrier added to their misery.

The decline in the medical services was explained soon after in an unusual meeting. I was looking for an apartment, and was approached by O. P. Edwards of the Hong Kong Bank. O.P., as he was called, gave me the address and an appointment to look over a flat which was owned by a Chinese general. That there might be some language difficulty only occurred to me as the elevator took me to the tenth floor. A "boy" dressed in a servant's long white gown opened the door and ushered me into the lounge where a small Chinese in a grey gown sat behind a desk.

"General Lim?" I asked.

"Ah," he said, "Edinburgh University Athletic Club, I see. I should have put on my club tie too." My necktie was distinctive, two diagonal stripes of different greens with small thistle emblems, the thistle being Scotland's floral symbol.

"You know Edinburgh?"

"I not only know it but we are fellow graduates. I was a lecturer in physiology under Sharpey-Schaffer."

"I apologise," I said. "O. P. Edwards told me nothing about you except that you are a general."

"Typical of Phil," he remarked. "He is my son-in-law."

Robert Lim had returned to China in the thirties and had rapidly ascended through the strata of official ranks to become Chief Medical Officer of the Chinese army; when we met he was also Minister of Health.

"I don't suppose you noticed the two tough-looking characters at the front entrance. Chiang Kai-shek knows I want to leave China, and he also knows that the Communists have broadcast over the radio, offering me the post of Minister of Health, so these two characters follow me everywhere. Chiang wants me to go to Canton and work from there, but this surveillance is very unpleasant. When I leave Shanghai I shall certainly lose this apartment which I own. If a foreigner rents it there is some chance of keeping it, so you would be doing me a favour."

40

We talked about the plight of the army and its wounded soldiers. All organised army medical care had more or less collapsed, but Lim was hopeful that China south of the Yangtze River would still be held, and was busy trying to reorganise the medical services.

Chiang Kai-shek was based in Chungking with the Nationalist armies during the war, and maintained an uneasy relationship with Mao and Chou En-lai. The Nationalists kept a fair proportion of their forces ready for action against the Communists, so their forces were not whole-heartedly committed to fighting the Japanese invaders, whereas the Communists persistently fought. Equipment, including medical supplies flown into China from India, arrived in Kunming and Chungking. Robert Lim insisted that, as the Communists were doing most of the fighting, they got their fair share of the medical supplies.

The Americans tried to get the two Chinese sides to join up to form an effective whole. From time to time Chiang and Mao cooperated, at least on the surface. Lim got to know both Mao and Chou En-lai who were grateful to him for his impartiality.

At the start of the Sino-Japanese war, O. P. Edwards was with the bank in Swatow where he was interned in the Foreigners' Club. As was fairly common in small towns, Swatow was under the control of the civil or consular corps of the Japanese, as opposed to army control. Internees tended to be treated much better under civil control officers, but although treated with relative lenience, the internees were not well fed and were perpetually hungry which drained them of energy.

Unfortunately for O.P., the Japanese consul developed a great interest in tennis. Lying on his bed after a meagre lunch, O.P. would be disturbed daily by the arrival of the consul's clerk who would solemnly bow and utter just one word: "tennis". He had then to get up and proceed to the tennis court where the consul was waiting. It would not have been so arduous if they had played normal tennis but the net had disappeared, and for two hours O.P. had to retrieve tennis balls from all over a couple of courts to hit them towards the consul, who then smashed them back without any particular attempt to return into the confines of the marked court. It was no good hitting wide of the consul; he would not run more than one or two steps, and such a stratagem resulted in O.P. having to retrieve the balls from the opposite end as well as his own. He came to dread the arrival of the clerk with his "tennis" summons.

The club also sported a nine-hole golf course. One morning while O.P. was sitting in a chair after a meal which was an apology for breakfast, the clerk appeared and bowed.

"Golfu," he said.

It was then that O.P. made up his mind to escape.

Before O.P. had been interned he had befriended an Armenian Jew who lived in the town of Swatow. Occasionally the internees were allowed into Swatow for shopping. This privilege was to be withdrawn but on the last occasion O.P. met the Armenian in Swatow. They faked a vicious quarrel supposedly over a debt and, marching off round a corner, rapidly made their way to the Armenian's house. There O.P. was introduced to the cook. The cook's position in the household was a cover, for in fact he was the leader of a gang of smugglers. With complete impartiality the gang smuggled Japanese goods to the interior; rice, a strictly rationed commodity, was carried on the return trip. The cook apparently approved of O.P. and agreed to set up an escape operation.

The Armenian visited O.P. on Double Island, an island in the harbour where the foreigners lived and had their houses. On the selected night the Japanese were informed that there would be no smuggling as it was a Chinese holiday and the tides were unpropitious for vessels to make their way up the Chiu Tung river. The Chinese holiday coincided with a Japanese festival, so the crews of the patrol craft were only too happy to have a night off.

The smugglers' boats were quite frequently apprehended by patrol craft; however, as their seniors were paid off the traffic went on merrily as long as things were not overdone. It was one thing for an inspection to reveal Japanese goods or sacks of rice, but totally different to find an interned foreigner lurking on board.

All internees were suposed to be in bed by nine o'clock when the electricity was cut off. That night O.P. went to bed with his clothes on, got up at 9:15, climbed through the window, and skirted the tennis court to reach the small jetty. There a sampan waited with two complete ruffians in charge and off they set up the harbour. At one point O.P. flashed a torch with a shaded beam in an effort to identify a passing structure as he feared that he might be in the process of being delivered to a Japanese shore station. This action earned him a blow across the back with a wooden club so he deemed it wiser to resign himself to his fate.

After two hours he realised he was up river from Swatow. The sampan pulled alongside a pier and O.P. was conducted to a nearby shanty. Inside were a group of men, the toughest-looking bunch he had ever seen. The black cotton garments worn by the Swatow waterfolk, seen in the faint light of a lantern, added to the sinister atmosphere. With great relief he recognised the man who got up to greet him — the cook-boy of the Armenian. They gave him the finest meal of fish and rice he had ever tasted. Later that night he was put on a sailing junk which took him farther up river where by morning he was handed over to a guerilla group. Some very hard walking for three days ended in O.P. being delivered to a mission group.

From there he went by truck to Kweilin, a place often depicted in Chinese paintings where the uniquely pinnacled hills rise from the banks of the river to dominate the landscape. Seventeen British soldiers, escapees from Hong Kong, were there and the party travelled by truck to make a record nineteen-day trip to Chungking.

O.P. told me that the varieties of human activities and character were well illustrated by the reaction of the different individuals in the party. They were each given the equivalent of fifty pounds sterling by the escape route organisation. Some of the men spent it in an orgy of whatever alcohol they could find and in whorehouses. Others arrived in Chungking three weeks later with the money still intact. The senior officer, a doctor in the Royal Army Medical Corps, Major Scriven, went to a local tailor who knocked him up a magnificent uniform in a couple of days. Nobody in Chungking knew exactly what army Scriven was supposed to be in. It bore a faint resemblance to a British Army outfit but also had a strong motif suggestive of an Austrian Hussar officer of the early nineteenth century. Scriven was proud of his uniform, and it was widely admired in Chungking by one and all until General Carton de Wiart, Winston Churchill's representative, caught sight of Scriven wearing it. De Wiart was a character himself, a Victoria Cross holder from World War I, and well known for the black patch he wore over one eye. Scriven was ordered into his office and told that if he was ever seen again in that uniform in Chungking, he would be court-martialled and probably shot.

At Kuosang the party made its last night stop before Chungking. There, in a spacious house at a formal dinner, O.P. was placed next to Effie, the daughter of General Lim and his Scottish wife. Had O.P. been sent on from Chungking to India to join the army, the girl might have slipped from his memory, but the Hong Kong Bank decided that, having a member fortuitously in Chungking, they would open a branch office. Phil and Effie met again and were eventually married.

One of the generally accepted concepts of banking is the possession of money and the willingness, under circumstances favourable to the bank, to part with it. Added to the difficulties of getting premises was the fact that there was no money to dispense. The opening of the branch was a typical Anglo-Chinese compromise. The outside was adorned with paper flowers and strings of crackers were exploded. Precious supplies of drinks were available for the distinguished guests, who included Madame Chiang Kai-shek herself. Each Chinese guest made a substantial deposit of cash; by the end of the party the bank was in both business and funds. O.P. went to bed happy but his joy was short lived — all the Chinese withdrew their money the next day.

Life was not always easy for the partners in a mixed marriage. One of my closest friends is Jack Huang. His father was one of the first Chinese to obtain an engineering degree in Britain, and had married a Scots girl from Glasgow. The relations in Scotland cut her out of the family when she married and went off to Peking, where her husband, Huang, worked on the Chinese Eastern Railway. It cannot have been easy for his wife in the early years of the twentieth century to be taken to Peking where there would be a marked prejudice against mixed marriages, both from the foreigners and the Chinese.

When her three sons were in their teens, Mrs Huang took them back to Glasgow to school. They called themselves Young while there, becoming quite well known in the suburb where they lived. Happily the Rintoul family in Glasgow relented, to accept them all back into the fold. The name Young was a convenience; when they returned to Peking they reverted to Huang and as such they remain today.

I first saw Jack when we were playing rugby in Shanghai. He was the opposing scrum-half. After the game I was curious to find out how and why a Chinese was playing.

"Och aye," he said, feigning a Scottish accent. "Ye come from the wrong side of the country. Did ye no play rugby for Watson's College?"

"Yes, what about you?"

"Kelvinside Academy where they taught us to play properly."

AN ESCAPE

Kelvinside Academy was in Glasgow.

Jack was one of the most even-tempered men I ever met. He was a good golfer, and would have been first class except that he never learned to chip. His golfing companions, of which I was one over many years, watched tensely as he lined up to chip or pitch onto the green. He almost invariably flubbed it: the expected happened and we doubled up with laughter. He is the only golfer I have ever known whose bad shots were greeted with real enjoyment by his partner and opponents alike. He would look up with a stunned expression of disbelief. A momentary flicker of irritation at the sight of our glee would flit across his features, but two seconds later he was laughing as heartily as we were.

Chapter 7

AMETHYST AND CONSORT

A surprised Amethyst fights back — A flight to Nanking — Consort at maximum speed, running the gauntlet — A diplomatic pass — The wounded arrive in Shanghai — Lt. Weston is spirited away — Amethyst makes the dash to freedom.

The uneasy truce between the Nationalists and Communists was finally due to expire at midnight on the 21st April, 1949. This affected the Royal Navy who, by agreement with the Government of China, had ships in several ports along the China seaboard and had maintained one at Nanking. As HMS *Consort* at Nanking was running short of supplies, the plan was for her to be relieved by the frigate HMS *Amethyst*, which left Shanghai on the 19th April to sail up the Yangtze to Nanking. The process of relieving ships had been going on for several months, including the three months when the Communists held the northern bank with the Nationalists dug in along the southern bank.

At about nine a.m. on the 20th, *Amethyst* was some sixty miles from Nanking when she came under heavy artillery fire from the Communists. Surprised, *Amethyst* nevertheless fought back but was heavily stricken and eventually ran aground on Rose Island close to the southern bank. The doctor on *Amethyst* was killed early in the action and her captain died later from his wounds.

HMS *Consort* set off from Nanking, making two efforts to range alongside and take the *Amethyst* in tow. She too came under heavy fire, sustaining many hits. When one hit damaged her steering she had to abandon the relief and set off down river for the mouth of the Yangtze and the China Sea.

I was sitting in my office when a man from the Consulate came in. He told me briefly about what was known and asked if I was willing to fly to Nanking and go to the *Amethyst* from there.

In the early afternoon I was at Lung Hwa airfield boarding a US Air Force B-25, known in the RAF as a Mitchell. I sat in the right hand seat alongside the pilot. The sun shone out of a cloudless sky on the green fields of the delta as the plane climbed away. After half an hour we picked up the broad, brown, Yangtze river, navigable by ocean-going ships for five hundred miles past Nanking to Hankow.

Flying at a couple of thousand feet, the peaceful scene unfolded with our progress. We could see the trench systems, gunposts and strongpoints of the Nationalists on the bank. At intervals of a few miles a gunboat was moored close to the southern bank. They looked very unwarlike with their guns at rest and not trained northward; washing was strung above the decks.

Suddenly a vessel appeared in midstream. From her crosstrees on each side flew a great white flag, and from her foremast a long white pennant stretched tautly aft beyond her stern, held stiffly by the speed of her going. It was the destroyer *Consort* going at maximum speed. Seldom does a destroyer work up to full revs in peacetime, and never in a river. A magnificent bow wave creamed back as far as the bridge; the wash spread in broad white lines across the muddy surface to crash far astern onto the banks. Her guns fore and aft were pointed hard to port, flames and smoke erupting from them. Great splashes rose in the river. An occasional explosion erupted on the south bank from an overshoot, but most of the shell splashes were several hundred yards astern. *Consort* was doing the impossible — running the gauntlet of a narrow channel against hostile, hidden, shore batteries, unable to turn or manoeuvre. All she could do was to cram on every ounce of speed, and fight back at guns unknown until they opened fire. We circled two times, saw the blue sky, green fields, grey destroyer with her foaming bow wave, dazzling white pennants, angry red gunflashes, shell splashes, black smoke streaming back from the funnels and the yellow water of the Yangtze.

I thought of her commander on the bridge, the gunnery officer laying her guns, the crew working like fiends, the engineers hammering her engines to near breaking point.

The starboard wing of the Mitchell swept up to the vertical. I saw the pilot holding the stick hard over as he executed a violent diving turn to pull out almost at ground level.

"The aim of this mission is to get you to Nanking, doctor, is it not?"

"I guess so."

"That little bit of aerobatics was when the bullets started to hit us," said the pilot, pointing to some holes which had appeared in the wing.

We climbed and picked up the river again where it made a bend to the south. There was *Amethyst*. She lay with her bow aground, listing to starboard. She seemed to simmer in the sun, motionless, out of action, crippled, a total contrast to the destroyer. The pilot said we would make one pass. Turning away to gain height, he came round in a circle and put the nose down heading for *Amethyst*. There was no one on deck, no one looked up or waved. Then she was gone under the belly of the aircraft.

The Mitchell braked to a stop in front of the control tower at the empty Nanking Airport. As I shook hands with the pilot he said to me, "Well, you and I are the only guys around who have ever seen that sight and I reckon we are the only ones who ever will."

A jeep took me to the Embassy where the naval attaché, a captain, asked me what we had seen.

"*Consort* was terrific. I could see no signs of damage or any hits. Most of the shell splashes were miles out."

"Great," he said. "We think she should be all right. She is well past the place where they started firing on *Amethyst*."

I was wrong. *Consort* had received many hits, mostly in her upper works. Fortunately most of the shells were incorrectly fused and many went right through without exploding.

We went out to a truck where a colonel was standing. He showed me the medical supplies and equipment loaded on it. We were climbing in when a sergeant ran up. The Communists had started to cross the Yangtze some twenty-four hours before the expiration of the armistice. We all went back into the Embassy and stood around conferring in the naval office. It was decided to abandon the attempt to reach *Amethyst* as night was approaching. The chances were that the attempt would fail and as likely as not both sides would start firing at us. A message had come from *Consort* to say she had many wounded and that she was proceeding to Shanghai. All those present thought I should go back by the first night train before the line was cut.

The naval attaché took me to his house in the Embassy compound where his wife gave me afternoon tea, and a jolly good tea it was — scones and jam, gingerbread and spongecake. Had she lit the fire, we might have been in a fine old house in an English shire. It was then I remembered that my passport was in Shanghai.

A diplomatic pass was issued to me; for a hectic two days I held diplomatic status. It certainly worked wonders at the station as I managed to procure a two-berth compartment. The thought that the train might run into the middle of a battle kept me awake for some time, but when sleep came it was sound. With some relief I realised on waking that the train was passing through a Shanghai suburb. Any ideas of breakfast, a bath and a change of clothes were dispelled as a junior consul hailed me from the platform before the train had properly stopped.

"You are to go to the dock right away. *Consort* is due in," he said. "A car is waiting." Sure enough, *Consort* was being warped alongside; jagged shell holes and shattered gear marked her whole length. Bennet, the ship's surgeon-lieutenant, met me. We already knew each other. His normal ebullient character was absent, his face showed a grey, drawn, mask of fatigue. At one point he was actually dressing a thigh wound when a shell passed right through the sick-bay removing the leg at knee level. The wounded were in several places — the ward room, officers' cabins; the sick-bay was a shambles.

"Look, Bennet," I said. "I know you have just about had it but you know who is badly injured. Can you organise them into the ambulances? Just scribble a label and tie it on to each saying when they last had morphine or anything else that is relevant; I had better go to the Country Hospital to start organising things there."

There were only Thorngate, Smolnikoff, and myself of our group in Shanghai at that time. One of the things which surprised me then and still surprises me in retrospect was the immense difficulty of sorting out a large number of injured men, deciding what to do and in what order. We received a lot of help from other doctors but the decisions were mine and I performed all the surgery.

Consort had been met in the river by the cruiser HMS *London* and the frigate HMS *Black Swan*; they had intended to reach *Amethyst* but came under devastating fire; both turned back with their quota of injured to land them in Shanghai. During that day and the next, the wounded from *London*, *Black Swan* and *Amethyst* started to arrive. The wounded from *Amethyst* were those that were fit to travel, and few were seriously hurt. The more seriously injured were in small, local hospitals one or two hundred miles from Shanghai. Between operations I had a quick look at the newest admissions and altered the priority list if necessary.

Going home for a brief half hour for a wash and change of clothes, my wife was relieved to see me, although the Consulate had kept her informed of my whereabouts as soon as they had found out anything definite. She was told that I had caught the train and fortunately did not know that the Communists had started their river crossing. Our second child was due to be born in two months so Jean had plenty to worry about.

From time to time on the second day a messenger would appear at the door of the operating theatre to say that another case was coming from *Amethyst* or had been admitted. I would break off and go to the open door to hear what had to be said. By the second evening the operations were easy, mostly finding and taking out pieces of shrapnel. As I was searching gently with a probe for the feel of metal in the depth of a thigh wound, another messenger appeared. Gowned and masked, I broke off to speak to him.

"You were issued with a diplomatic pass," he said. "I have been sent to get it back."

"I don't happen to have it on me," I replied.

"Where is it?" he said, horrified. Obviously some thought went through his mind that it had been flogged, possibly to a spy.

"It is in my trouser pocket at home."

"I'll go and get it."

"No, you will not," I said. "I shall bring it here tomorrow morning when good and ready to do so." Thus ended my diplomatic career.

Grandiose plans had been made against the coming of the Communists; the plan was to concentrate the British population at Holt's Wharf during any hostilities. The presence of a Royal Navy cruiser alongside the dock was an essential ingredient of the plan. After the treatment meted out to *Amethyst* and *Consort*, the plan more or less collapsed totally; but before it was officially scrapped it was obvious that it must be scrapped. From the office window I watched the last Royal Navy ship, the frigate HMS *Black Swan*, slip her moorings to slide slowly downriver to be lost from sight round a bend in the river. This sight gave me what might be described as "that sinking feeling". The lifeline had been severed.

It was now imperative to get the wounded out of China. Some were put in ambulances, others climbed into trucks; the small convoy drove off to the dock to be loaded on a landing craft. Each man held his somewhat scanty medical documents. As one or two of the men were missing a limb and others were far from well, some expression of anxiety, some aura of depression might have been expected, but they were as cheerful a bunch as you would find anywhere. If it were not that some were on stretchers, they might have been supporters of the football team that had just won the Cup. Such men were there on the China station because they had either asked to be there or had not asked not to be there. All forty-four of the wounded who had been treated in the Country Hospital went out in the convoy. They all survived. I would like to think that it was due to my skill, but in honesty I must attribute this to their youth, fortitude and resilience.

Not all of *Amethyst's* wounded had reached Shanghai before their crewmates were evacuated; some who had been in small hospitals, too ill to travel, continued to arrive for over a month. One of these was Lieutenant Weston, who came in one day, a month or so after the Communists had taken Shanghai. An X-ray showed an impressive chunk of metal in his liver. This foreign body he considered he could do without, but whatever X-ray view was photographed, the three by one inch shadow always appeared bang in the middle of the screen. The dark metal shadow seemed to stay in the same place when the rest of his anatomy moved around it. Surgery of the liver was not commonly done in 1949.

"Lieutenant," I said to him, "that thing has been in there for several months. It was red hot and bacteriologically sterile when it went in. It is doing you no harm. Just keep it there till you get back to England where one of the boys who specialises in liver surgery can advise you. We don't have the back-up services here anyway."

I think Lt. Weston was pretty bored doing nothing instead of pacing the deck of a warship. He was in a sort of limbo, not officially being in China at all. Partly just for something to do in the mornings he would drop into my office to discuss the matter of his steel holdings, a matter which I would again dismiss before we talked of other things. He always said that he would be cooped up in China for ages because the Communists did not view his predicament with sympathy. After *Amethyst* excaped from the Yangtze his position became even more tenuous.

I realised one day that I had not seen him for some time and was missing his cheerful visits. He had been spirited away and although it would have been indiscreet and futile to have asked how, there is no doubt that the Yellow Ox Gang must have been in the deal. This large Chinese secret society still flourished for a year or two after the Communists arrived on the scene. They could still get people out at a very big price.

A year later in Hong Kong, while thumbing through an old *Illustrated London News*, I saw a full page photo of the *Amethyst* crew in a ceremonial march through Plymouth. Slap in the middle of the first row, smiling, looking fit and cheerful, was the stocky figure of Lt. Weston. As he habitually looked fit and cheerful, I could not judge from the picture if he was still in the scrap metal market.

Commander Keran took over *Amethyst*, conducting stealthy repairs, and when all was ready she made her dash down the Yangtze to freedom. This was front page news in the *North China Daily News*. As she had fought her way, the propaganda machine pulled out every stop. Criminals, murderers, bandits, the fire breathed right out of the newsprint. We were jubilant but the jubilation was mixed with a chill foreboding.

When you and your family and friends are aliens and virtual prisoners in a land with a hostile regime, a shiver of apprehension in bed at night is pardonable as you contemplate what reprisals, organised or individual, may fall upon your persons. Most British like ourselves were wide-awake long before the newspaper, a sad shadow of the former independent *North China Daily News*, was delivered. I was standing outside the door waiting for the delivery boy. Grabbing the paper from him, I looked at the front page with trepidation. There was no mention of the *Amethyst*. I tore through one page after the other, but there was nothing. It was never mentioned again. The foreign community was almost as astounded by the lack of news and repercussions as by the headlines of the day before. But news travelled fast and by lunchtime the mystery was solved.

It appeared that long after *Amethyst* had passed in the early dawn, the Woo Sung forts had opened fire on an innocent Chinese ferry setting off on its lawful business across the wide mouth of the Yangtze estuary. The batteries had sunk it with considerable loss of life. The captain had climbed ashore very indignant indeed, had come back into Shanghai, and shouted his story, so to speak, from the rooftops. When a tremendous mistake has been perpetrated, when the consequences have been dire indeed, when slapstick has reached a zenith, the Chinese ache with laughter. It was the funniest thing that had happened for six months and the population were starved of humour. In embarrassment the propaganda machine clammed up.

My own theory about the reason for the shelling of *Amethyst* in the first place stems from the picture in my mind's eye of the Nationalist gunboats moored with an air of permanence along the south bend of the Yangtze. The Nationalists had already made a deal with the Communists to be taken over, and when *Amethyst* steamed

AMETHYST AND CONSORT

up river (remember that the Communist troops had probably never seen a warship in all their lives) they went into action assuming that an agreement was being flouted.

53

Chapter 8

WE ARE LIBERATED

The end of an era for Shanghai — A night in a police station — The currency outruns the supply of banknotes — The Communists silently enter Shanghai.

By the beginning of May 1949 it was clear that the end of an era for Shanghai was approaching. The Communists were advancing slowly and remorselessly; brave statements were made about defending the city street by street, but it was evident from day to day that authority was collapsing. However, the sheer difficulties of living occupied so much time that lawlessness neither increased nor became a factor worth considering. The hour of curfew, at first midnight, crept slowly forward against the clock. Police action became more summary — shoot first and then ask questions. One broke the curfew at the risk of a rifle shot.

One night, having visited the hospital, I sped home with ten minutes to spare before the curfew; outside the gate of our apartment block a police officer stopped me to ask me to give him a lift to Zikhawei police station. As he was cradling an automatic pistol, it was wise to accede to his request, so in he got. When we drew up outside the police station he glanced at his watch, and said to me, "You are out after the curfew — inside." My remonstrations were brushed aside as I reluctantly followed him in. While the recipient of my kindly, albeit choiceless, good turn for the day disappeared into an office. I was brought up sharply at the reception desk to register. My protests were totally ignored and I joined the other delinquents sitting on the hard floor against an equally hard wall. I was allowed to telephone home to tell Jean where I was, and not to expect me back till dawn. About four a.m. another protest was registered at the desk, to be greeted by a curt nod indicating that I could be on my way. But at the gate the police sentry thrust his rifle through the open window of the car; he had not been briefed, so back I marched to resume my place on the floor, which now seemed harder than ever. At six a.m. the fifty or sixty arrested, having paid a fine, were released *en masse*; my misfortune was finally recognised because no subscription to the police on duty was asked of me.

The currency was now slipping so fast that it had completely outrun the supply of banknotes. Silver dollars and ounces of gold were peddled in certain streets, and authority woke up to the bright idea that these semi-illegal coins and gold bars could be changed in special exchange shops. Repairing to a nearby exchange shop to change some dollars for notes to purchase our day's supplies, I found a motley crowd waiting their turn. Suddenly the door burst open and two smartly dressed men of the "Special Police" came in. Both were big, tough, ruthless men and were carrying machine pistols. One pointed his gun at the ceiling and ripped off two shots. The roar of the firing was followed by a dead silence; the smell of fear instantly permeated the room. Then both men guffawed and barked out an order. Moving slowly along the lines of customers, they laughingly removed about half of each man's money except for one man whose offering was meagre. He got a pistol butt crack on his chest which persuaded him to find a lot more cash in his pockets, of which he was promptly relieved. When the police came opposite to me, one nodded his head at me as though we were old friends and passed me by. They swaggered out, stood on the pavement obviously looking for the next shop and we resumed trading. There was no uproar; we had just accepted the inevitable.

Our apartment was on the tenth floor affording a view over the northern suburbs of Shanghai. After dark, in the quietness that descended with the curfew, the guns would start firing. I could not decide if they fired during the day. Possibly the sound was lost in the roar from the city, but it was likely that in the stillness the sound had more impact. Certainly the tracer shells created shafts of colour as they streaked out to the north; after all the target was big — the whole of North China. The firing was a reminder to the citizens that a crisis was approaching.

The plan for the concentration and protection of the British population, under the umbrella of a cruiser at Holt's Wharf across the river, collapsed. This was succeeded by a more modest operation. Everyone would stay in their houses except for small groups of young men who were armed with clubs or staves to guard the Club, the Country Hospital and a few selected properties. The Club was the nerve centre forming a headquarters for what it was worth.

As Burton and Smolnikoff lived right by the hospital, I was stationed at HQ. When it was obvious that the city would be taken either that night or the following night, I repaired to the Club.

Hardly had I settled in before a phone call came from the hospital to say that one of the guards there, Ian Gauntlet, had in the course of his duties developed a right-side abdominal pain with fever and vomiting. Burton told me to come on over and take out Ian's appendix.

It was eerie to drive along streets which had always been filled with traffic and bustling crowds but were now completely deserted; all the shops had their shutters down. Not a soul was outside except for sentries stationed at large intersections and the occasional military patrol. It was nervous work driving very slowly, coming almost to a halt, hoping thus to convince the soldiers that my business was both lawful and without malice. The soldiers looked at the car with interest but showed no signs of hostility; however, because one group did nothing it did not mean that the next would act likewise. It was with considerable relief that the car stopped for the hospital gates to open.

Although not more than three hours had elapsed since Ian's first symptoms, his appendix had already perforated by the time it was exposed. It must have been one of the fastest developing cases of appendicitis on record, giving rise to a good deal of ribald comment subsequently because of the infection which dragged on for almost a month. A surgeon who does not cure such a short-lived disease with expediency is judged to have made a mess of things. "After all," was the comment of one of our mutual friends, "he was in the hospital when it came on. Wasn't he?" Ian slowly recovered; he was a popular figure, later killed when the Spitfire he was flying for the Hong Kong Auxiliary Air Force plunged into the sea.

Rather than return to the Club, I made my way carefully back to our apartment, and Jean and I visited neighbours in other flats in our apartment block. The tenseness increased with an almost tangible quality as darkness fell. The city was in almost total darkness, as a light might attract some hostile action. We returned to our apartment. Suddenly the telephone bell rang.

"Hullo," said a voice from a bachelor's mess near Hung Jao on the outskirts of Shanghai, "they are coming past the house." Lines of men were padding softly along the road. "They are absolutely quiet; have they reached you yet?" Most people had expected some sort of noise but the Communist soldiers wore soft-cloth boots so that even the crunch of soldiers' boots on the tarmac was missing. We indulged in a good deal of peering out of our darkened windows till about midnight, when I called my secretary who lived two miles farther out. She also was looking out and had received progress reports from her friends. Nothing was happening, so there did not seem much to do except go to bed. Sometime in the night there was a single long burst of machine-gun fire outside on the street. In the morning a few people could be seen walking along the road. I took the lift down to the hall and saw some five or six Communist soldiers sitting on the steps tucking into bowls of rice ladled out of a large pan. We stared at each other with silent appraisal. At the nearest intersection on the street there was one soldier at each corner cradling a rifle, totally ignoring the few pedestrians. A battered old Nationalist armoured car sat abandoned with its machine gun pointed skywards; the crew had obviously fired off all the ammunition into the night before leaving it.

We had been "Liberated".

For a day or two following our "liberation" there was a degree of resistance. Soochow creek had been the dividing line between the old International Settlement and Chapei, where the Chinese had put up a bitter two-month resistance to the Japanese in 1938. A force, mainly of Taiwanese, together with troops who were essentially Chiang Kai-shek's personal guard regiment, held the creek and bridges against the Communists, who kept up some light arms fire in a drawn-out skirmish. There was no need to mount a full-scale attack with heavy weapons as a strong force could easily outflank the position to make it untenable. There were bullets whizzing about up and down the streets, a fact I ascertained by phoning a couple who lived in a flat on one of the roads involved.

"Old Smith," I said over the phone, "wants me to make a house visit. He lives just round the corner from you."

"Well," replied the husband, "all the downstairs windows are gone and a machine gun opens up at regular intervals from Nanking Road, and there are one or two bodies lying about."

I called Smith who corroborated the information, sounding very surprised that as a doctor I had not been issued with a pass guaranteeing me immunity.

"The Nationalists did not give me one and I have not had time yet to get one from the Communists." After a pause I added, "Yet," hoping thus to convince him that as soon as this was obtained nothing would stop me intervening personally in the war.

Smith bore me a grudge thereafter. One of my friends told me he kept muttering about the Hippocratic Oath, but in that worthy document there is neither injunction nor obligation for a doctor to drive his car and disembark therefrom on a street where two angry armies are firing at everything that moves. Smith, it may be added, recovered spontaneously and without medical treatment from whatever it was that was afflicting him; it was, as far as I remember, low back pain, known in those bad old days as lumbago.

The Nationalists pulled back from Soochow creek to embark at Woo Sung near the mouth of the Shanghai river. Their withdrawal was marked by a pall of black smoke drifting over the city from the firing of the oil tanks at Woo Sung; this last sign of their going burned slowly for a day. People started to move about but there was never the same bustle, the same activity, the same energy, the same gaiety; the pulsating life of Shanghai with its colour, excitement, spontaneity and charm was gone.

Chapter 9

LIFE UNDER OUR NEW RULERS

The Shanghai Ice and Cold Storage Company and their eggs — Foreign firms are milked of their assets — The Hessian and Gunny Bag Dealers hold a farewell dinner.

The breakdown of authority, the inefficiency, corruption, tension and venality of the last months of the Nationalists impelled a belief that any change would be for the better. There was a longing for stability of government; it was thought that under a just, steadfast regime, opportunities for trade would be restored. True, trade and industry would have to be accomplished under different rules and guidelines. These prospects were fostered by firms or agencies who indicated that the Reds were principally agrarian reformers, rather than Marxist influenced.

Apart from the large, old-established trading firms called *hongs,* mainly British, many other organisations with international reputations and world-wide interests had a large stake in China, involving trading, factories, equipment and property. These corporations hoped not only to preserve their holdings but also to renew activities which were beneficial not only to themselves but to China. Oil companies, bankers, insurers, textile manufacturers, importers and exporters, charitable organisations, missionaries and religious groups were amongst a host of enterprises with interests and capital locked up in China.

There were many unique organisations geared specifically to the China trade. For example, such an organisation with a division devoted totally to a parochial business was the Shanghai Ice & Cold Storage Company. It was true then and it is still true today that the Chinese devote more time to the preparation and cooking of food than any other race, including the French. Strangely, although chicken is an important dish, by some quirk of culinary aberration the Chinese neither value nor prize the humble egg. Before the turn of the century, some astute foreigner realised this and over the years built up an enormous business. As long as there was water transport and collecting depots, small farmers and peasants were only too willing to be paid for a commodity for which there was little demand.

The peasant's wife, by selling a few eggs, earned a copper or two for what was barely a useful item. The eggs were delivered from a million sources, preserved in ice as soon as they reached a small depot, and collected on junks and sampans to be brought down river to Shanghai. The eggs could only be sufficiently fresh and in commercial quantity if the collecting system cast an enormous net into the hinterland with a widespread batch of agents.

On arrival in Shanghai the eggs came into the factory. There, scores of girls sat at tables; in front of each girl was a metal prong embedded in the desk. The eggs came past her on a moving belt; she took an egg, broke it on the prong, smelt it to make sure it was fresh and if so, emptied the content into a four-gallon tin. If the egg was bad she threw it behind her into a refuse trough. One bad egg ruined the content of a four-gallon tin. When one considers that prewar there were special refrigerated ocean-going freighters whose only cargo out of China to Europe consisted of tins of eggs, it will be realised that literally billions of eggs arrived in Shanghai. Eggs and egg powder used in baking in Europe depended almost entirely on this source. Such a trade could only benefit the Chinese people.

By 1949 the collecting system had begun to work again; it had taken over three years to get it going. Thousands of far-flung agents earned a small income from a part-time activity; thousands augmented their pay from being involved at an intermediate level; hundreds in the depots and transporting sections depended on the trade; and finally there were large numbers processing and packing in Shanghai. The Ice & Cold Storage Company rightly concluded that such a trade, depending on a few cents profit at its multitudinous origins and gradually building up like a pyramid towards the centre, could only flourish in an environment of free enterprise, no matter how minute that enterprise might be at its origin.

A variety of sources, including the British Embassy, had fostered the "agrarian reformers" theory and had encouraged me to stay in China. "You will be in on the ground floor" was a favourite expression. Shanghai was a turbulent city with a higher proportion of entrepreneurs than anywhere else. With its history and tradition of free trading, its population were less inclined to the Marxist theories and more independent than in other cities. Furthermore there were the largest number of such people in one spot. It behoved the Communists, therefore, to pay lip service to this spirit. A hard-fisted tyranny would play into the hands of a powerful, truculent opposition and indeed, for the first month, life was much better than before. The faint shadows then began to appear; slowly at first as control became surer, and then faster and faster until control was absolute. Then the grip was all embracing. Stories crept around of arrests, people disappearing in the night, school children informing on their parents. Each street had its commissar who watched and reported. It became obvious that hopes of trade and individual enterprise were gone forever. Some foreigners left and more were about to go when the Nationalists dropped mines in the Whang Po. All shipping ceased; we were not trapped, just locked in.

The Communists then proceeded to milk the foreign firms by taxes, by supporting workers' claims, by forced trading at a loss, by one means or another. Everyone who had ever worked for a foreign firm appeared claiming wrongful dismissal even if they had worked only for a brief time many years before the war. Houseservants were amongst those who appeared demanding three months' pay for every year of work, which later increased to a year's pay for each year of work. When this became utterly ridiculous, the authorities did not say the employee was wrong, but they took most of the payment as tax. House servants rapidly reduced their demands to one month's pay per year, which was more or less the standard accepted in the bad old days. One large firm, which was paying out vast sums to real and bogus former employees, discovered that it was faced with a charge of wrongful dismissal by two employees whose funeral expenses the firm had paid for only a year before when the two men had been drowned in a ferry disaster. The firm took the matter to court exhibiting photos of the funeral from the Chinese newspapers. Even the Communists balked at the claims and arrested the impostors, but the report in the newspaper said that the firm had "confessed and apologised for its errors".

Businessmen underwent very marked unpleasantness. The authorities backed up the workers' claims, and businessmen were locked up in their offices all day and half the night. To make a concession resulted only in whetting the appetite of the workers for more. In desperation a businessman might appeal to a tribunal, in which case an official sat at the top of the table, obviously in sympathy with the workers, and showing indifference or antagonism to the businessman. Some of these sessions were convened daily for months. Every now and then there would be a mild triumph. As all the employers compared notes they eventually constructed a strategy which worked with varying degrees of success.

Shanghai Ice and Cold Storage had a remarkable success owing to the fact that the authorities wanted to recreate their business with the eggs to earn foreign exchange, but the Communist doctrine is such that it could not be admitted that the foreigner had any justice on his side at all. The *taipan* or manager of Shanghai Ice had been told that he would have support, but the charade had to be played out; he too was engaged in daily confrontation with his workers, but the official in "the chair" showed a lack of the usual sympathy with the workers, who realised that they were not doing nearly so well as workers in other tribunals. They eventually lost their tempers and shouted that they had been better off under Chiang Kai-shek's regime. The official rose to his feet and declared the meeting closed; the tribunal was reconvened after a day or two but the workers' representatives were not the same men. The originals were never seen again. The Chinese are people who believe in fair dealing; the workers in the tribunal sessions were the militants, but many a foreigner was encouraged by expressions of sympathy from the moderate vast majority — a word here, a smile there or merely an overt gesture.

It was, and still is, the official line that the foreigners exploited the Chinese. There is, of course, a great deal of truth in this, but they were exploited a great deal more by their own kind. Generally speaking, any Chinese who worked for a foreign firm was paid much more, was advanced if he was worthy, and might well prosper hugely. Furthermore, apart from schools and universities instilling direct learning, the trades introduced by foreigners bred a class of mechanics and technicians at all levels, a class of clerks, bankers, and insurance men. The Chinese who worked with and for foreigners were envied by their fellows. It was not a one-way benefit.

Being an employee myself, and the only doctor in our group who was not a partner, I was not above gently hinting, when occasion demanded, that I was another of the world's workers with my face being ground into the dust to satisfy the avaricious demands of my ruthless employers. These sentiments, lightly brought up without being too specific, eased my path when I was eventually arranging to leave China.

One group of traders, the Hessian and Gunny Bag Dealers Guild of Shanghai, read the writing on the wall with commendable speed. Middlemen were on the way out fast. The Guild decided just three weeks after "liberation" to dissolve in haste. No doubt the members benefited from a financial division of the spoils, reserving a portion for a final dinner. The members were all Chinese but over the years, indeed for the best part of a century, they had dealt intimately with Jardine Matheson & Company's subsidiary, the Ewo Cotton Mills. They invited Ronnie Gosling, the Jardine's representative, along to the function, advising him to bring another foreigner of his choice to join in the celebration. He asked me to join him.

Most Chinese are abstemious where drinking is concerned but the Hessian and Gunny Bag dealers proved exceptional to a man as far as I could judge. Looking across the huge top floor of the restaurant, the windows gave onto the broad, green expanse of the former race course. The function was in full swing when Ronnie and I got there at around six in the evening. Bottles of Black Label Whisky, only the best, were emptied at alarming speed. We sat down at about seven as the first course was served. It was a feast. Course after course appeared, spread out over three hours. Our glasses were never emptied except to drink a toast; the eating was only interrupted three times, firstly for a speech by Ronnie, both his eloquence and his Chinese stimulated by the fare. He indicated right away that the Gunny Bag dealers were a crowd of brigands, that they had consistently over the years cheated Jardine's, that their double-dealing and rapacity had caused him personally great distress, but he was sorry to see them go. This speech was a tremendous success, and we all drank to these sentiments. After a suitable interval for another course, the Dean of the Guild got up to welcome Ronnie and myself. He went on to explain that Ronnie and his firm, Jardines, had been hard taskmasters, that the foreign devils had ground every cent and drop of sweat from the honest Hessian men, and had made a vast profit, that they had never paid a fair price for good articles and sold inferior rubbish to the dealers. It was a wonder that the Guild had survived. Everyone drank to this with wild enthusiasm. The noise level, aided by noise from the two lower levels coming up the open well staircase, reached a crescendo. The success of a Chinese dinner is directly related to the din created. Judged by such a standard this meal gained top marks.

Opposite me sat the Dean, corpulent in a Chinese gown. He was totally bald, with a sun-tanned scalp. His great round face creased as he smiled and laughed; he was a sort of cross between Buddha and a successful warlord. Some dealers were fat, others very thin, but all were dressed in Chinese gowns. Jolly rather than handsome, they all had that look which made one think it would not be wise to cross them, but that fair dealing would find them firm friends. Four of them took Ronnie and me off to Del Monica's nightclub, grabbing a bottle or two on the way. There were still some taxi-dancers, so called because you bought a ticket for each dance with the hostesses there. The nightclub was closing in the following week because guests were scarce. As far as I remember, and things were getting a bit hazy, we shared the attentions of some twenty or more of the girls who may not have looked much in the light of day but on that night looked marvellous. It was the end of the era of taxi-dancers and supple, slim hostesses dressed in tight-fitting *cheongsams* split at each side to reveal provocative glimpses of knee and thigh.

Many of the foreigners would have left China had it not been for the mining of the river. About a year went by before they were allowed to leave by going to Tientsin in North China by rail and there catching a ship. In that year, by one means or another, they were successfully milked of what assets they had. Mine were sparse to begin with but I contributed my share. The method used was to put a tax on an asset such as a club; all members would contribute to keep the facility going. Three months later a much stiffer tax was imposed and as soon as the deadline was met a still greater tax was immediately levied. In lieu of the tax, the grounds and buildings would be handed over, but only after the signing of a document stating that the handover was done willingly and without coercion. Businesses and property went the same way, except that a businessman, on handing over his business, was subject to an additional closing down tax. Being victims of their own propaganda about the ruthless exploitation of China by foreigners, such methods seemed only fair to the authorities.

Chapter 10

A BOMB HERE AND THERE

"Pushface Gin" is launched — The scuttling of a river steamer — A lumbar puncture under unusual circumstances.

For several months after the taking of Shanghai we were entertained by Nationalist planes dropping bombs on targets carefully selected to avoid alienating the population at large. By the time this activity became organised, one's sympathies were with the attackers. We had moved to a top floor flat of a ten-storey block of apartments in the Western district. The roof provided a grandstand view of several raids. Because the anti-aircraft fire was totally ineffective the bombers came in line astern on slow, accurate run-ins. The explosions at Lung Hwa airfield were quite spectacular; the most impressive raid was a mid-afternoon affair against the electric power station. Some twenty four-engined heavy bombers flew a steady course at about four thousand feet, putting their bombs slap on the target. From the flames and smoke it was obvious that the power station was receiving a large number of direct hits. We had a fine view and derived some satisfaction from the performance. Our pleasure did not last long, ceasing abruptly the moment I pressed the button to summon the elevator. Nothing happened. The lift was at the fourth floor and there it remained for three weeks until our enterprising landlord installed a motor car engine to generate current and even then it only ran at certain hours. The thought of climbing to the tenth floor dampened one's ardour for going out. We had friends on the second and seventh floors; seldom, if ever, did we make the climb without two rests for refreshment on the way. As alcohol was getting in very short supply it was politic to augment our friends' supplies in order to make sure that we were welcome.

The whole foreign population was beginning to suffer from a severe shortage, when Ken Hall of the Duro Paint Company came to our rescue. Up till that time I was not aware that alcohol was an essential ingredient of paint. To maintain paint production, the factory was allocated a generous supply of grain alcohol. Ken as manager was able to siphon off a small quota of the precious fluid from which he prepared a respectable gin, which for some reason he called "Pushface Gin." It was first launched at a Saturday luncheon of a married couple who had a house with a large garden. Some hundred people milled around the lawn consuming the gin in considerable quantities. The guests were heartened firstly to acclaim its smooth, delicious taste and secondly to be assured that there would be adequate supplies. The tasting and assessment were so thorough that lunch was postponed until the sun was going down behind the trees. Jean and I returned to our apartment at about seven in the evening, to go to bed before eight and sleep soundly till after nine on Sunday. Some of the more persistent guests stayed till late on Saturday night. Most of them slept for eighteen hours; one man slept a full twenty-four hours. Pushface Gin was withdrawn for further refining. The new product was carefully tested for its soporific effects by trial and error rather than chemical analysis, to reappear on the market for fairly select clientele. It was only sold by the Winchester or half-gallon bottle at a ridiculously low premium. Ken Hall did not want to be accused of profiteering, despite supplying what amounted to a basic ingredient of life itself. Paint in commercial quantities apparently consumes vast quantities of alcohol; the diversion of a hundred thousandth of the supply did not dent the economy of the People's Republic which found out about it, fortunately for Ken Hall, after he had departed from China. The firm had a very sticky time of it, being accused of sabotage, subversion, deviationism, and other serious crimes all rolled into one.

Apart from the large air raids, individual planes had a habit of appearing over the city in the afternoons; this kept everyone on their toes. The planes usually focused their attentions on craft in the river to avoid injuring friend and foe alike. These activities involved a minor crisis at Drs Marshall, Jackson and Partners when a chunk of shrapnel came sailing through the open window, hitting the ceiling before landing on Victor Smolnikoff's desk bang in front of him. He reached forward to pick it up, not realising that although it was not actually red hot, it was hot enough to blister his fingers and thumb. It was then decided by the partners that the downtown office should be manned by the assistant in the afternoon. We were all presumably expendable but the assistant just happened to be more expendable. As trade had diminished to a trickle or indeed vanished altogether, after lunchtime the only men still around the business section were juniors like me; they were young and healthy and would only visit a doctor from boredom so the work was not onerous.

A BOMB HERE AND THERE

By going out onto a small balcony one could spot hostile air action, and retreat under cover when an aircraft seemed to be almost overhead. In some ways this was preferable to sitting in the office wondering if a bomb would come through the roof; outside, looking at the sky, the period of anxiety might never develop if aircraft were obviously not coming right over the top. Usually the aircraft were twin-engined Mitchells, or B-25s to give them their American name. Occasionally a single engine fighter did a job on its own; one of these did a most spectacular dive over the river, releasing a single bomb which hit a tugboat going on its lawful business. The direct hit sent up a spurt of flame from the tugboat's bow, but the tug continued moving forward, going down very rapidly by the head. Two figures scrambled up the deck to climb onto the stern, and both dived into the river as the stern suddenly plunged straight downward beneath the water. The curious thing was that the figures did not jump but dived neatly and gracefully. Both of them swam ashore right below my balcony. Without warning or previous training, they had suddenly become the wettest men in Shanghai.

A more leisurely, slower process was taking place on the near bank a couple of hundred yards along from the office window. A river steamer had been scuttled. Masts and funnel lay under water, but part of the decks and half the hull above water pointed toward the Bund. Salvage operations got under way, the first problem being to get her upright. A group of concrete bastions were constructed on the shore. Huge hawsers passed from the concrete anchors over raised pulleys and across the vessel to be attached to the submerged side of the hull. When the four or five hawsers were in place, a series of winches started working to pull the craft upright. The newspapers carried photographs and articles explaining that socialist ingenuity and know-how backed by the thinking of Karl Marx was about to achieve a success which was utterly beyond the skill of capitalists, handicapped as they were by the absence of Karl Marx's blessings. After about a month of preparation the winching started; by the evening of the first day she was at an angle of about 45°, and the masts and funnel were well clear of the water. Unfortunately, I did not get down to the Bund office till late the next afternoon but then I hurried to the window. Like the sex machine in the vulgar song we sang as schoolboys, "There was no means of stopping it". The riverboat, presumably having been pulled upright, had not stopped but toppled over in what would have been a complete port to

67

starboard arc except that the masts and funnel, now bent out of kilter, were resting on the Bund, preventing the full half-circle turn. The matter rested there for a while. No doubt the engineers were doing a bit of brushing up on Marxism before further efforts. The second time round, they succeeded in righting her, without benefit of publicity.

The defences, of course, had a considerable number of guns which blasted away with great enthusiasm without achieving anything positive except to injure people with bits of shrapnel. Anti-aircraft guns were not installed in the urban area, but machine guns and 20 mm cannons sprouted on roof tops. One of the fastest lumbar punctures ever was performed because of these cannons. The patient, Jones, was an Eurasian ship's officer, although I imagine he was not qualified and did not possess a mate's certificate. He obtained work on coastal craft, tugs which did ocean-towing contracts and other odd seafaring jobs. Unfortunately for him he tried to get a visa to Australia as a refugee just too late; his Wasserman reaction indicated a syphilitic infection. Although he had received more than adequate treatment he fell into the category of one whose blood test would not revert to normal. Today, as long as certificates of full treatment are provided, I believe the irreversability of the blood test is accepted, but in 1949-50 authorities were reluctant to accept this, and furthermore would require a negative Wasserman test of the cerebro-spinal fluid.

Because Jones was "on the beach" and stony broke, I arranged to do a spinal tap in the office rather than the hospital, thus saving him the hospital expense. The skin of his lower back was anaesthetised with local, and he was sitting upright with his legs over the side of the operating table. I put the point of the lumbar puncture needle and stillette against the skin, and gave it a small thrust to penetrate the skin. Normally one then holds the needle at the correct upward angle, advancing it slowly and carefully strictly in the midline, hoping to push it gently through the aperture between the spines into the spinal canal. Even doctors who do this frequently often do not hit the aperture first time — the needle point comes against bone, and has to be withdrawn slightly to alter the angle.

I had just got the point through the skin when there was a deafening, shattering roar. No one had told me, much less Jones, that a 20 mm cannon had been installed on the roof right above our heads. The snarling rip lasted only a few seconds but it was enough to make both Jones and me do a sitting jump. I looked at the needle — it was in about three or four inches.

"Hold it! Hold it!" I shouted and withdrew the stillette; cerebrospinal fluid dripped from the needle. Having grabbed a test tube to start collecting the fluid, another burst of firing caused us to jump again. The fluid still came out, and when there was 10 cc in the test tube I yanked out the needle. To consider that I hold the world's speed record for doing a lumbar puncture is presumptuous but I reckon I must be in the top ten. Happily for Jones it was all a great success; firstly he did not suffer the headache which may follow a spinal tap especially if the patient does not remain recumbent, and secondly his cerebo-spinal fluid showed a negative reaction. He got his papers to become an Australian citizen. A few years later two gigantic clam shells found off some South Pacific Island were delivered by a seafaring friend to my office in Japan in token of his gratitude.

Next day, Jean said to me over lunch, "I am sure I heard a jet aircraft this morning." Sure enough, the next day I saw three MIGs hurtling across the sky. The bombing came to an abrupt and complete halt.

Chapter 11

THE INDIAN CONSUL

Shipping the Sikhs out of Shanghai — Millin's Prostatectomy creates near panic — The long and tedious task of unravelling the riddle of a name.

The International Police of Shanghai before the war had several hundred Sikhs, who became unemployed with the end of extra-territorial rights. Most had no education with nothing to contribute to the community; the best they could do was to fulfil the jobs of watchmen or caretakers. They existed on the borderline of starvation in conditions of squalor. Their homeland became part of the new India, so the Sikhs became the responsibility of the Indian Consulate. They were a major thorn in the flesh of Mr Uppal, the Indian Consul.

Mr Uppal was a small, rather dapper man who strove unceasingly to alleviate the lot of the Sikhs; his ultimate grand design was to ship them back to India. Depressed by poverty, the Sikhs nevertheless got supplies of liquor which led sometimes to fierce quarrels and extreme violence. When a Sikh ran amok with a knife or club he did a very thorough job on one of his compatriots. Owing to some quirk in the Indian consular procedure, it was necessary to have a certificate stating that death was the result of an attack. The certificate could not be from a Chinese police surgeon, but had to be from a doctor of a friendly power. One glance was enough to confirm that the death of the victim had indeed been violent.

On two separate occasions, my telephone rang in the early morning and Mr Uppal introduced himself to explain that he would be obliged if I would come down to help out with a rather nasty accident. My suggestion that the accident case be sent to hospital would bring a guarded remark to the effect that the predicament would not benefit from hospital care. I proceeded downtown and took the elevator up to Mr Uppal's flat where I was greeted by him and a vice-consul.

"Doctor," Mr Uppal said, "as you know, we Hindus do not drink alcohol but the circumstances are so horrifying that we must make an exception and brave ourselves to witness this unpleasant

70

business," whereupon he reached under his desk to bring up a bottle of Black Label. A glance at the bottle revealed that Uppal and company were about to fortify a resolve which had already been subject to remedial treatment. He then poured a half tumbler for each of us; under the circumstances it was not judged to be necessary to dilute the medicine with water. Strong measures must be taken to give us strong nerves.

On the first occasion we proceeded to a shack, and on the other to a mortuary, to view the remains. Without doubt, the scene was spectacular; both corpses had up to a dozen frightful wounds, any single one of which would have been fatal in itself.

"You are prepared to certify that he died violently?" asked Mr Uppal with a touch of anxiety, in case I were to consider that the man had died from natural causes. Having assured him that the certificate would be appropriately signed, we trooped back to the car and back to the flat where the certificate was ready for my signature. Before I was asked to steel myself to sign the document, we all had to partake of further concentrated therapy which emptied the bottle.

Eventually Mr Uppal, a conscientious and persistent man, persuaded the Indian government to charter a small liner to ship the Sikhs back to India. His efforts were even more praiseworthy because the ship did not come into Shanghai until after the Communist takeover. Not only was it one of the first vessels allowed in, but it managed to get in just before the Nationalists mined the river.

We were all involved in the flurry of inoculations and all the arrangements to transport the physically handicapped and so on to the dock. The police were glad to assist as the authorities were only too happy to be rid of a small but troublesome group of aliens; the whole community were rounded up to embark on the ship. I had forgotten that it was "D" day for Mr Uppal until I happened to be walking along the Bund and caught sight of his small, neat figure coming toward me. If it had not been for the Bank of China building, Mr Uppal would not have been progressing at all. With every second step he staggered, cannoning off the wall as he went along. He recognised me when we were a few feet apart and came to a swaying halt.

"Every one," he said, "every one of them, every one of them ish aboard and she hash started. No more trouble with dead bodies; no more, no more." The bottle of Black Label he had taken to the dock had seen Mr Uppal through another harrowing experience. Little did he realise his troubles were not over. When they reached Hong Kong, all but a few jumped ship, and the vessel proceeded to India almost empty.

The Indian Treasury and Foreign Office seemed to consider that Mr Uppal was personally responsible for wasting a lot of government money and bore down on him with a series of very nasty reprimands. Personally, I thought Mr Uppal had done a very fine job and I hope that in the long run his meritorious service in difficult circumstances was recognised if not rewarded.

It is one thing to set out to retrieve a surgical case in a desperate condition; quite another to create such a condition. At a surgical conference a young Chinese surgeon asked me if I would like to give him a hand with a Millin's prostatectomy. Millin had pioneered a new method of removing the prostate gland; he had published a record of his method in considerable detail, but at that time my only knowledge of the procedure had been gleaned from a highly favourable general article in the British Medical Journal which did not, however, go into the details of the technique — the specialised instruments used, after-care procedures and hazards. I presumed that the Chinese surgeon had studied the surgical publications, and had probably seen the procedure done. Chia, my driver, after stopping to make enquiries, eventually deposited me at the front door of People's Hospital No. 5, somewhere in the depths of the suburb of Chapei. The surgeon took me straight to the operating theatre where we proceeded to "scrub up", prior to donning operating gowns. While working with the soap and nail brush I became aware of a tall, stern-looking man right behind me, quite literally breathing down my neck. I turned to look at him, to receive a steady stare which frankly had all the markings of hostility. The Chinese surgeon scrubbing up at the next basin saw the querulousness of my expression.

"He is the Communist official in charge here," he said. "Don't worry, he has no English at all."

"Has he any medical knowledge? "I asked.

"No. He is just the Party man."

"Difficult customer?"

"He can be," replied my companion. The first twinges of anxiety flitted briefly across my mind, but the surgeon changed the subject.

"You have a driver?" he asked.

"For me it is absolutely essential. Imagine what would happen if I ran over a Chinese."

"I see what you mean. What do you pay your driver?"

I told him.

"He gets more pay a month than I do."

There did not seem much to say to that, although I could well believe him.

When we got started, it soon became apparent that the surgeon was expecting me to do the operation; there was some polite discussion about this and I managed to persuade him that I had no desire to usurp his prerogative, so he proceeded. It was soon very obvious that he knew even less about the technique than I did. We soon ran into some really spectacular bleeding, but this was not a matter for serious concern, because we could easily deal with it. But then I became aware of some very heavy breathing in my left ear and the presence of a large man leaning against me to peer over my shoulder. The feeling of anxiety returned in an acute form. It was not necessary to look around to realise who it was nor to sense that disapproval was mounting to create a situation where some dramatic action might result. Possibly I was totally wrong in my assumption. The Comrade may just have been evincing a layman's interest, and my visions of ending up in front of a hostile tribunal the result of some preconceived notion, but finally I was in a state of near panic. It does not take long, a few seconds only at such a time, for the panic to spread. We floundered on for a few more minutes; things were getting worse and worse.

"I think," I said, "we had better abandon the Millin's and go back to the routine method I usually use." He readily agreed so I took over. By any method, prostatectomy is a bloody business; in fact, the control of the bleeding which must occur is the crux of the operation.

Most surgeons detest the presence of lay people at an operation. Normal behaviour is altered, and there is an additional strain. Panic is the worst thing that can happen. In certain cases one can, of course, explain to a lay person what is going on, why you do this or that. With a sympathetic person you may well be at ease, but with a suspicious representative of an alien ideology holding your fate in his hand, one of the most unpleasant situations arises. Everyone in the theatre was aware of this, not least the Commissar.

My confidence slowly returned. In the end it was not a difficult case at all; the difficulties were of our creation. When it was all over it was a tremendous relief to sit sipping tea alone with the surgeon and interns. We did not mention our mutual friend who, no doubt, was busying himself elsewhere in the hospital making sure that things were being done without any deviationism whatsoever.

With this case I trusted no one. Telephone calls did not satisfy me. Chia and I seemed to spend most of our time travelling to Chapei and back. Morning and evening found me paying a visit. If the Commissar was not at the front door when I got there, he showed up immediately. He trailed me along the corridor and into the ward, never once nodded in recognition, did not reply to my "Good morning". A nasty piece of work he was.

About two weeks later the case was discharged. I never saw the patient again, I never went back to the hospital, never saw the surgeon and, best of all, was never again subjected to that presence at my shoulder or the piercing satanic look. I had learned a lot of lessons all rolled into one. I also sent to my bookseller in Scotland asking for a copy of Millin's monograph.

My family name used to be Maclagan Wedderburn but, as Wedderburn is a big enough mouthful in itself, my father and most of his generation dropped the Maclagan part of the surname, although we retained it as a given name. When Jean and I were married she adopted it as a given name. She registered with the immigration authorities as Jean Maclagan Wedderburn, but somehow the Maclagan was missing on her passport.

A policeman, selected to unravel the riddle by dint of his knowledge of English, arrived at our flat. However his English was so rudimentary that he was quite incapable of understanding anything at all complex. We realised that he had been a policeman under the Nationalists, merely changing his uniform to conform with his new masters. His rank was lowly and likely to remain so no matter whom he served. We wrestled for an hour with the problem of the discrepancy between Jean's registration and her passport, without getting anywhere. Mr Chen, the shroff, was asked to come to the flat the next evening and all was explained in great detail. Mr Chen went on to hint that with the capitalist system this sort of blunder was all too common and regrettable, and that such errors would not take place under an enlightened system. Furthermore our gratitude for exposing the matter to the light of day was boundless. The policeman took copious notes.

The next evening he was back again so we went through it all again; Mr Chen reported for the second time on the fourth day exercising tact and patience. A break occurred over the weekend but Monday found our friend again ensconced in the lounge, and he was there from about five to seven p.m. every evening for six weeks. He did not say so but there is no doubt that his superiors did not accept the explanation. As the thing had been thrashed out over again and again he did not bother to raise the questions.

We rearranged the furniture so that his chair was offset from the mainstream of lounge activity; our cook gave him a cup of tea, and he sat warming his hands at the fire. At first Corinna, our daughter, attempted to play with him, offering him her dolls and toys but as his response was lukewarm she soon found better things to do. Apart from nodding to him when we came in, we ignored him as he gazed moodily into the fire. At about seven he would get up and leave without a word.

It was obvious that he was not doing too well with his enquiries but any sorrow we felt because of his predicament soon turned to indifference. Sometimes we speculated that he might be merely turning up to get warmth and relaxation but ruled this out on thinking of what would happen to him if the suspicion of fraternisation were raised.

To have suggested that we ourselves go to the police, a thing one would have done in a democracy, was not even considered; such action might well bring down coals of fire upon our heads.

In one way we benefited from his presence, and he became something of a "cause celèbre". A constant stream of friends dropped in during the evenings to view the phenomenon. As he could not understand anything but the simplest, slowly and carefully enunciated English the handicap of having to muzzle opinions or topics did not exist.

"How's Charlie Boy this evening?" someone might ask.

"Much the same, possibly a bit more morose than usual."

Things might have been a lot worse if his English had been good. We should have had to censor our remarks in case he reported our lack of reverence for the new authorities. This was another reason not to complain; we might have been saddled with a sharper character who devoted part of his time to listening for "wrong thinking"; even the most innocent of remarks could easily be misinterpreted and twisted. Under similar circumstances a Chinese family would have suffered agonies of apprehension. Then one day he just did not turn up, and was never to be seen again.

75

Had he convinced his superiors? Was he sent off on a course of study? Was he promoted or demoted, reprimanded or praised? It remains one of life's minor mysteries.

Chapter 12

WE DECIDE TO LEAVE

The foreigners close ranks — Physicians have a field day with parasites — Old and new fractures come to our attention — Misadventure on a river steamer — We prepare to leave Shanghai.

Two months after the start of the new regime, the honeymoon was coming to an end. As the weeks followed, it became more and more obvious that there was going to be no place whatsoever for a foreigner; even the few fellow travellers were neither welcome nor able to penetrate the blank wall which greeted their gestures of friendship. A large exodus of foreign residents took place when the SS *General Gordon,* half passenger, half troop ship, entered the port to embark those who had arranged to leave. Many foreigners like ourselves had judged it necessary to do likewise but when the Nationalists mined the river, the exit door was slammed. The foreign community drew together, in adversity becoming bed fellows. The large firms, such as oil companies with a huge stake in China still nominally in their charge, banks, insurance companies, and big trading *hongs* all had their quota of foreign employees.

Another curious feature of belonging to a minority was the suppression of nationality. Under a hostile administration with so many problems in common, English-speaking foreigners formed a brotherhood which included other nationalities such as the Dutch and Scandinavians who were all fluent English speakers. I have lived in other communities in the East where one is always aware that a person, no matter how close a friend, is not, so to speak, "one of us". This type of awareness became totally submerged in the peculiar circumstances of being free but still confined. The whole community felt as one when a Scots youth, slightly inebriated, and driven by some petulant urge, left his apartment and took a rickshaw to Party headquarters in downtown Shanghai where Chen Yi, a hero of the Long March, had his headquarters to govern Shanghai. The Scot dismounted, and to the total astonishment of the two armed sentries, reached into the rickshaw, took out his bagpipes, blew them up, started to play and marched straight through the front door. He climbed two lots of stairs, went through various offices, down back through the front door and got into the rickshaw. As far is it was known no enquiries were ever instituted, although the boss of his firm had him on the mat the next day. Probably dear old Lenin had not covered this contingency in his writings.

Smolnikoff too, despite his selection of ideology, remained a firm part of the foreign community, firstly because he was very popular and secondly because for several months the Russian Consulate, with some Slav perversity, continued to be ultra-correct by still recognising the Nationalists, thus placing Smolnikoff in a sort of limbo. Large numbers of Russians from Russia appeared in the city. Some were technicians but most were thinly-veiled members of their armed forces. They supported the newly created Chinese air force, artillery and other specialised military units. There was no truck between the Russian home-grown products and the Shanghai exiles even if the latter had opted for Soviet citizenship. For the year we were there, Smolnikoff was still used from time to time by the Consulate. Sometimes he was pressed into helping the other indigent Russians but there was no meeting between him, his like, and the exported variety of advisers from Mother Russia. In some ways the Chinese authorities were more suspicious of the converted than the out and out capitalists; authority knew where it stood with the latter.

Our practice had diminished in numbers, leaving Burton, Smolnikoff, Yieh, Thorngate and myself. Most of the foreigners were under "contract". Employees were guaranteed their medical expenses while abroad; the contract was a fixed sum per capita which allowed the person to have office visits, home and hospital visits, an annual physical examination with chest X-ray and some laboratory tests. Surgery, X-ray, and so on were charged separately. This was a satisfactory arrangement both from the patient's point of view and from that of the employer who would pay a set sum twice annually for the medical care of all his staff. The doctors in turn could budget knowing that certain fairly substantial payments would be made at regular intervals. Some of these contract payments were made to a bank in Hong Kong in foreign currency. Eventually this illegal procedure led to disaster.

Although our pool of patients diminished during the first few months until the mining of the river, it was augmented fairly regularly by individuals arriving in Shanghai from anywhere in the Yangtze valley. Trading companies closed down in distant cities and the employees were pulled back into Shanghai. Missionaries, priests and nuns arrived in a steady trickle. It was surprising to realise that there was a sprinkling of foreigners who had retired in the remotest areas of China. A man who had a small workshop carving curios from a special stone found in a remote valley, a Belgian or American who had cultivated a farm in the back of beyond, scholars studying local customs, culture or hieroglyphics — all manner of men who had chosen to live in totally alien surroundings, driven by some inner urge, happy to cut themselves off entirely from the environment and companionship of their birth and education. Many were now forced to give up a lifetime's work, most were either penniless or had sold their few assets for a song. Quite a number had long neglected medical conditions; now, with nothing to do, they got their haemorrhoids, varicose veins and hernias put right. The physicians had a field day finding a multitude of parasites — liver fluke, lung fluke, round worms, tape worms, hook worms, and parasitic diseases with exotic names like Kala Azar and Schistosomiasis. Nobody enjoyed himself more than Hsieh, our laboratory technician; he was often seen scurrying down the corridor to a doctor's office bursting with the news that he had run to earth some fascinating egg recovered from the gut, some object showing a characteristic changing shape while it still wriggled on a microscopic slide. We all peered down the microscope at these bizarre discoveries, nodding our heads sagely, swiftly going back to our office to reach for a book to find out first what it actually was, secondly how to treat it. A quick perusal of the treatment often convinced me that the hazards were the province of physicians; surgery has enough of its own without taking on others. For instance, a book I still have deals with bilharzia; introducing a typical physician's rhetoric, it says "Sodium Antimony Tartrate (Tartaremetic) first successfully used by Christopherson in 1917 still retains pride of place — Intravenous injections of *freshly* prepared solution are given on alternate days starting with ½ grain and working up — dependent on the reaction — to 2½ grains, till a total of 30 grains has been administered. The drug is exceedingly toxic both locally and systemically. Great care must be excercised to ensure that the venipuncture is accurate and that none of the drug is extravasated into the local tissue or sloughing of the tissue, destruction of the vein and a troublesome ulcer will result. The general toxicity of the drug may manifest itself by a cough, vomiting, giddiness, collapse, diarrhoea, jaundice, muscular pains and occasionally sudden death." Smolnikoff and Burton could keep their bilharzia cases to themselves and Thorngate could look after the lung flukes as far as I was concerned.

Yieh and I had our own "field day" with badly united fractures, some old, some fairly recent. There always had been a supply of these reaching Shanghai but previously most were recent, immobilised by inadequate wooden or bamboo splinting, the victim possibly having taken two weeks to get to Shanghai. But now a crop of very old fractures, completely united in very bad positions, began to appear. Yieh was very conservative in his approach. As the years have passed I realise just how wise he was. Meddlesome surgery is very wrong; the target must be mapped out very clearly and the possibility of achieving the target must be very accurately assessed.

Some of the folk attempting to reach Shanghai had a great deal of trouble. One of the joys of living in a Marxist state was the necessity of obtaining a permit to travel. One day a group of foreigners closed down their offices and set off on the few days' trip by river steamer from Hankow to Shanghai. The captain anchored for the night near the river bank in a large tributary which, as often happened, was in flood. In the middle of the night the travellers became aware that the vessel was listing. As their bunks gradually tilted, they got up to be told that the vessel was aground. By morning the list was very marked — they were tending to fall out of their bunks. By afternoon the steamer was high and dry in a paddy field. As another flood might not occur for months, the passengers hired coolies to carry their luggage and they set off across the fields to the nearest township where they were all promptly arrested and locked up in an inn for illegal entry into the province of Anhwei. The captain himself was not very happy, incompetence being not far removed from sabotage. The distrust with which petty officials in the regime greeted all such untoward incidents was given free rein. The captain had both to defend himself and to explain the predicament of his passengers who were immediately suspected of being spies, subversives, and opponents of the regime. After a frustrating five days with several difficult interviews they were issued permits to travel to Wuhu where all the interviews were repeated. Previously the stranded steamer was a piece of evidence to corroborate their story, but now the evidence was a hundred miles away. They were up to their necks in a sea of suspicion until, at last, train permits were issued to allow them to travel to Shanghai, where they arrived in good fettle, glad to be back in what amounted to civilisation.

Despite the influx of people from far afield it was obvious that there was no future for my family and myself in China. Just a month after the Communists took Shanghai, our second daughter, Alexandra, was born. In the spring of 1950 the railway to Peking and Tientsin in North China was reopened. All who were able to travel started making plans to leave. Unlike, for example, the employees of big companies, who knew that when their permits came through they would be re-assigned to jobs with their firms in other parts of the world, our problem was dual: firstly to get out and secondly, what to do then. It was not an enviable position to be a member of a disintegrating organisation. The income of Drs Marshall, Jackson and Partners was steadily falling. My pay, based on a realistic rate of exchange, was steadily reduced in real terms by relating it more and more to the official rate. Merely to live I had to bring back from Hong Kong the meagre sum that I had managed to save. It was not practical to complain too much. Burton had been interned for four years. The practice he had put together again after the war was once more falling to pieces; everything that he had worked for was going down the drain. McGolrick had had better luck. He was on leave in 1941 and had joined the British Army as a medical specialist, but he, too, saw his assets eroded to nothing. Thorngate had been interned at the beginning of the war but got out on an internee exchange ship to America. Yieh, being Chinese, was stuck but he was well qualified and later became the chief consultant for the whole Shanghai/ Nanking region. Smolnikoff was always broke anyway but he did not like it any better for that reason. In a way, with youth on my side, I was better off than any of the partners; at least I had prospects.

My plans to go to Japan, first suggested to me by the dentist John Besford, received help from several quarters. Curiously, at that time it was still possible to phone Hong Kong. I put through a call to Dr Jack McElney, who had been my host in Hong Kong when the Shanghai rugby team played there, and the call was indeed fruitful. I asked him for a temporary job while waiting for my entry visa to Japan. Jack was a real go-getter, who seldom sat still for more than three minutes. He told me to hang on while he went to see Dr Anderson, their senior partner and surgeon. Jack was back in a minute.

"Andy wants to go to Canada for four months. Can you be here by the first of July?" he asked.

"Yes. At the moment it is taking about two months to get an

exit permit."

"I can't tell you what we will pay you but you will be all right."

"Many thanks, Jack. See you before the first of July."

"What is it like up there? Bloody awful, I suppose."

"You're a hundred per cent right. Still, we are surviving."

It was settled.

Chapter 13

LEAVING CHINA

Going through the formalities of leaving — The necessity for certificates, documents, photographs — Packing with precision and papers — Smuggling gold in a bar of soap — Pushing papers for two coins — What befell the friends left behind.

The decision to leave China was one thing, going through all the formalities was another. Sometime about nine months after Shanghai was taken, although the river was still mined, the railway to Peking and Tientsin had been restored. Armed with the necessary permission one could travel by train to Tientsin and from there take a ship to Hong Kong.

The first step was to declare our intention of leaving. We were then furnished with a form like a small booklet. This was only the beginning. Eventually my exit permit carried fifty-three "chops", or rubber stamps. The shortest time that it took to achieve any one stamping was twenty minutes, and the procedure developed into a full-time occupation. During many interviews, obvious distrust and dislike were barely concealed. Only on two occasions was a spark of interest or humanity evinced; one was when Jean's jewellery was being valued by a Customs official in Tientsin, the other was in Shanghai when a clerk looked at our passport photographs. He could see from the picture that Corinna was a girl but Alexi, as we called Alexandra, was only nine months old. He asked if the photo was that of a boy.

"No," I replied, "she is a girl."

"I am sorry."

"Thank you," I said. "It is not so important for a foreigner to have a son as for a Chinese."

To have made even such an innocent enquiry in front of his colleagues was tantamount to fraternisation.

Documents and books were examined separately. When living abroad it is necessary to carry all sorts of certificates, letters, and papers. These were subjected to close scrutiny before being placed in the attaché case brought along for the purpose. The case was then locked by the owner and the official put the appropriate seal around it. Woe betide the owner should the seal be tampered with or broken; firstly, the suspicion of foreign subterfuge was raised and secondly, the examination would be repeated with greater and more prolonged probing. Several people who had not provided a good receptacle underwent this fate. It was all too easy to tear the seal because it consisted of a strip of thin, delicate rice paper. I carried the small briefcase cradled in both arms as though it were a time-bomb liable to explode with the slightest vibration. It sat on top of a cupboard in the flat until it received similar care on the way to the station; it occupied its own space on the luggage rack in the train. It continued to receive favoured attention in the hotel in Tientsin until finally we climbed the ship's gangway.

Jean carried another small case holding photographs and snapshots. These had been passed and inspected in a completely different office which used good strong seals. We took nearly all our photos with us although every one had been closely examined. Only two were removed without any explanation. I think, in fact, that this was purely a gesture on the part of the official to show that he was doing his job.

Books came in for inspection at still another office. Most people did not bother with books and these I kept to a minimum, but medical and surgical textbooks are expensive and difficult to replace. Mine were rapidly passed although as well as being flipped through, they were held up by the outside covers and shaken in case something loose was concealed between the pages. Sensibly enough the seal put on the small crate I had brought along was robust enough to withstand rough handling, and I do not remember having any anxiety on its behalf.

I cannot recall what many of the visits and chops were for; one of them, however, involved misgivings and unease. A notice had to be put in the newspaper for three days declaring the intention of the person to leave China, coupled with a warning to anyone who had any reason to object to lodge their objection with the pertinent bureau within seven days. No matter how blameless an existence one had led, it was impossible to eliminate some qualms when entering the bureau after the requisite interval. Most accusations were related to pay or unjust dismissal. For the most part these were dealt with fairly but they involved long interviews, and in borderline cases the foreigner paid. I did worry about the houseboy who had taken Mr Chen and myself to the police station, but neither he nor anyone else saw fit to implicate me in wrongdoing.

Then it came to packing. No commissary of a military unit, no supply officer of a mountaineering expedition, approached his problem with the care we did. Every item in every suitcase or crate had to be listed with six copies in both English and Chinese. Copies in English can be run off on a stencil or carbons, but Chinese does not lend itself to even one carbon copy; half the clerical staff in the office were busy for days painstakingly writing out copies again and again in neat legible characters. Stories filtered through from Tientsin of people getting in very hot water because there was one too many shirt in suitcase No. 6 or three too few handkerchiefs in No. 4. Everyone who has ever packed a case before travelling knows that as soon as the case is closed and locked, there is an immediate need to open it again. All these impulses had to be resisted; once cases Nos. 1 to 8 had been listed and closed they had to remain so. As all this listing took time, it had to be planned about two weeks before the date of travel, with trial packings of the cases still to be filled by the clothing or articles needed for day to day use.

Thorngate left a week before we did, so there were only Yieh, Smolnikoff and Burton to say goodbye to. There was an air of finality about our farewells, as we knew that it was unlikely that we would ever meet again. Yieh, particularly, was distressed. There still were some restaurants providing good Chinese meals, so on one of our last evenings he gave us a sumptuous meal. As we left to go to our cars he took my arm so that we walked apart from the other guests.

"You know," he said, "there is no future here for me unless I join them." It was his apologia.

I put an arm around his shoulders.

"Dear Yieh," I said, "you know that I understand."

During the last few months our staff began to leave. The regulations were such that anyone who left was substantially compensated, but there was not enough money to pay everyone. I had little option but to suffer a reduction in my salary. To live, even to exist, my meagre savings in a Hong Kong bank had to be utilised. It was still possible to deal through money brokers but because of the risk they ran their commission was formidable. All our furniture, our refrigerator and our household goods were sent off to an auction; at one point it seemed as though the costs of moving the furniture to the auction and the auctioneer's charges would be more than the value fetched by the sale. It was a relief to get about US$30 for the lot. It was particularly exasperating to have to sell the Austin car which had taken the place of the Model A. It was only twenty months old, and realised only US$60.

Some months previously, Archie Teacher of the China Soap Company, the subsidiary of an international concern, had sold me two ounces of gold. Each ounce formed a small rectangular bar which bore the chop of the goldsmith who had made it. Their value when I bought them was US$45. I asked Archie to sell them for me as they represented a high percentage of my worldly wealth.

"You don't want to sell them," he said, "you will only get US$25. Give them to me and I shall see what can be done."

A week later Archie saw me in the club. He took a bar of Lux toilet soap from one pocket and a second from another.

"Hold this one in your left hand, the other in your right. Don't mix them up — now tell me which bar holds the gold."

Weighing them in separate hands I could not decide.

"Put the one from your left hand in your pocket and give me the other," said Archie.

"Thanks, Archie," I replied. "You mean the gold was put in during the making of the soap tablet?"

"Yes."

"Can you trust the man who did it?"

"There is only one who knows. I can trust him."

During the customs examination on the dock at Tientsin I watched the inspector lift the Lux tablet from one side of the suitcase to the other as he rummaged through the case. I had no qualms, and I derived a great deal of satisfaction from pulling "a fast one". When we were safely at sea I found Jean had taken the soap from the case to use it in the cabin. The second time I retrieved it she became suspicious, wanting to know the reason why. When she was told, far from congratulating me on my skill and acumen, she dealt at some length on the stupidity of the risk I had taken. In Hong Kong, taking a sharp knife, I neatly bisected the Lux. It divided nicely into two halves. Alarmed, and cursing Archie's perfidy, I cut the halves in two. Fortunately for my peace of mind the first quarter yielded a solid resistance to the blade. Archie had offset the ounces in opposite corners.

One of the last formalities was the valuation of jewellery. Probably many of the men who had interviewed, questioned, and inspected us were ex-civil servants of the old regime, but in the company of colleagues with an inevitable cadre present they could not adopt any attitude except a stern one. However, when it came to the jewellery business we were alone with an old style Chinese who had been with the China Maritime Customs for many years. Precious stones were his speciality. We gathered from him that official policy was that the Capitalists — we felt flattered — deemed some jewellery as a requisite of life. The matter was condoned, although to be deplored.

We had a long chat with him. One of his tales filled him with a sort of benevolent sadness. The authorities were quite reasonable, provided that the number of rings, brooches, and so on was not excessive. If the suspicion was aroused that money had been converted into precious stones as a means to get it out of China, some or all would be confiscated. A certain number of White Russians were getting out of China. Facing an uncertain future in strange foreign lands they could be desperate and they had converted their often meagre wealth into stones; they suffered anguish if the jewellery was out of proportion to their other goods. The old man told us that an owner when asked what value he put on a stone, would for the most part quote about two-thirds of what he or she really thought. His smile obviously included us in this category. The White Russians, however, hoping for the best, fearing confiscation or the levy of export duty, would quote about a quarter of what they thought the value was. He referred especially to some of the young women who might have bought a diamond recently or received one as a present from some erstwhile boyfriend in the American services, for services rendered.

"If they say $500," he remarked, "I know they think it is really worth $2,000."

He looked at us solemnly, his expression suffused with sorrow as he contemplated human frailty and deceit.

"I have to tell them, 'It is a zircon, worth $5'."

Eventually we left Shanghai. Two days and nights by train took us across the large fertile plain of North China, over the Yellow River and into the foothills of Shantung Province. I could recognise the different shapes of the fields and the types of trees and crops, from my time as a schoolboy in Chefoo. The people too were taller and tougher looking than in the south. We spent two weeks in a hotel in Tientsin.

Most of my last day in China was spent in the Peoples' Bank of

China. Each foreigner was allowed a small sum of Hong Kong dollar currency for his use on the voyage. Having collected the allotment for the family, I produced two silver dollars. We had taken them along the day before for the jewellery inspection only to be told by our friend there that these were currency. The two coins had been given as mementos for Corinna and Alexi; one was a US dollar and the other a Chinese Junk dollar, so called because the emblem on the coin was a junk.

Having enquired regarding the possibility of taking these coins, a form was handed to me. A messenger-interpreter arrived on the scene and together we proceeded to a different counter. The need for the messenger soon became apparent. We went from one desk to another, up to the third floor, down to the first. The project got under way about nine in the morning. At noon we were standing before a desk we had been at twice before, awaiting a further rubber stamp on the form.

I asked the messenger how far along the line we were. The man behind the desk, who on our previous stops had conducted affairs through the interpreter, looked up to say in perfect English, "You are about half way."

"In that case," I said, "I am happy to donate these two dollars to the People's Republic."

"You have started the proceedings. You will finish them."

He was not quite right as it turned out. Using time as a criterion we were about two-thirds toward completion. At 2.15 pm I tottered down the steps clutching an export licence in one hand and the two dollars in the other.

They took the export licence off me the next day at the gangway of the SS *Hupeh*. I was all ready to give it an honoured place in my collection of secret and important documents. The silver dollars are still in our possession.

The *Hupeh*, a vessel of Butterfield & Swire, had accommodation for twelve passengers but we were crowded on board with some forty others. The passengers lined the rail and when the last rope connecting us to the shore was untied, a spontaneous communal sigh of relief was heard.

Over the years I heard what fates befell the friends I had left behind. For Tom Burton, Shanghai had been his life and he would stay on until there was nothing left for him to stay for.

One day, his office door burst open; two uniformed men pointed submachine guns at Miss Wong, the receptionist, and told her not to move. Miss Wong did not move. Two more men rushed down the corridor to the records and accounts office; in no time they had the book and papers with transactions of money paid into the firm's Hong Kong account. Burton was taken into detention but he was barely interrogated, merely shown the records from the office. In the evening, expecting to be moved to Ward Road Gaol, he was surprised when he was allowed to go home. During a quarter of a century Burton had helped many people in illness and in health, Chinese as well as other nationalities. Beneath his gruff exterior and glowering mien he had never acted dishonestly. He had aided and succoured countless people, wealthy and poor, true men and crooks, coolies and soldiers of fortune. Perhaps because of this, perhaps because of his artificial leg, or perhaps for some totally unknown reason, he was allowed home. An old Scots friend of his went round to Burton's house in the evening; the friend carried one of his two remaining bottles of Scotch whisky. They spent the evening together. One of the things the friend told me about the evening was that despite the fact that it was a warm night in early May there was a big fire burning in the fireplace because Dr Burton said he felt cold. Smolnikoff was called early next morning by the houseboy. Burton had had a stroke. He recognised Victor but could not speak. He died the next day.

Yieh became Chief Orthopaedic Consultant of the Eastern Region of China, and was drafted almost immediately into the army. He was sent to North Korea in control of the Orthopaedic services of the Chinese army during the Korean War. Knowing Yieh, he would not have enjoyed that one bit, but I have no doubt he did a very good job.

Smolnikoff stayed in Shanghai till 1953, then with his family he set off for Russia. He spent his first year working in Siberia not far from Lake Baikal. I received letters from him when he was doing what seemed unlikely in Russia, namely, in his own words, "Private Practice," in the even more unlikely locale of Samarkand. We wrote once annually until a time came when it was obvious that my letters were no longer reaching the correct destination. In the late 1960s, Sir Robert Mackintosh, the doyen of British anaesthetists, was lecturing in Hong Kong about his experiences on his recent trip to Russia. He said that one of Russia's leading anaesthetists had started on the ladder of anaesthetic prowess in Kiev, climbing the ladder to be a

Director of an Anaesthetic Institute in Moscow.

"The curious thing about this man was," said Sir Robert — in a flash I was hanging on to his words; I knew what he was going to say, but not the words he would use — "he had come from a firm of British doctors in Shanghai."

Finally I can think of only one benefit which accrued from our year under communism's red banner.

Owing to what was almost certainly a prodigious bureaucratic blunder, several railway trucks, which probably should have gone to some Russian town with the improbable name of Omsk or Tomsk, found their way to Shanghai. Vast quantities of caviar suddenly appeared in the markets, and soon a pound of caviar was cheaper than a pound of butter.

It was all too easy to become addicted and we are now lifelong addicts. There was so much that we fed it to our cat Rachael, and she loved it immensely.

Considering the ruinous price of caviar in the rest of the world today, I am not sure if this benefit is in fact a true blessing.

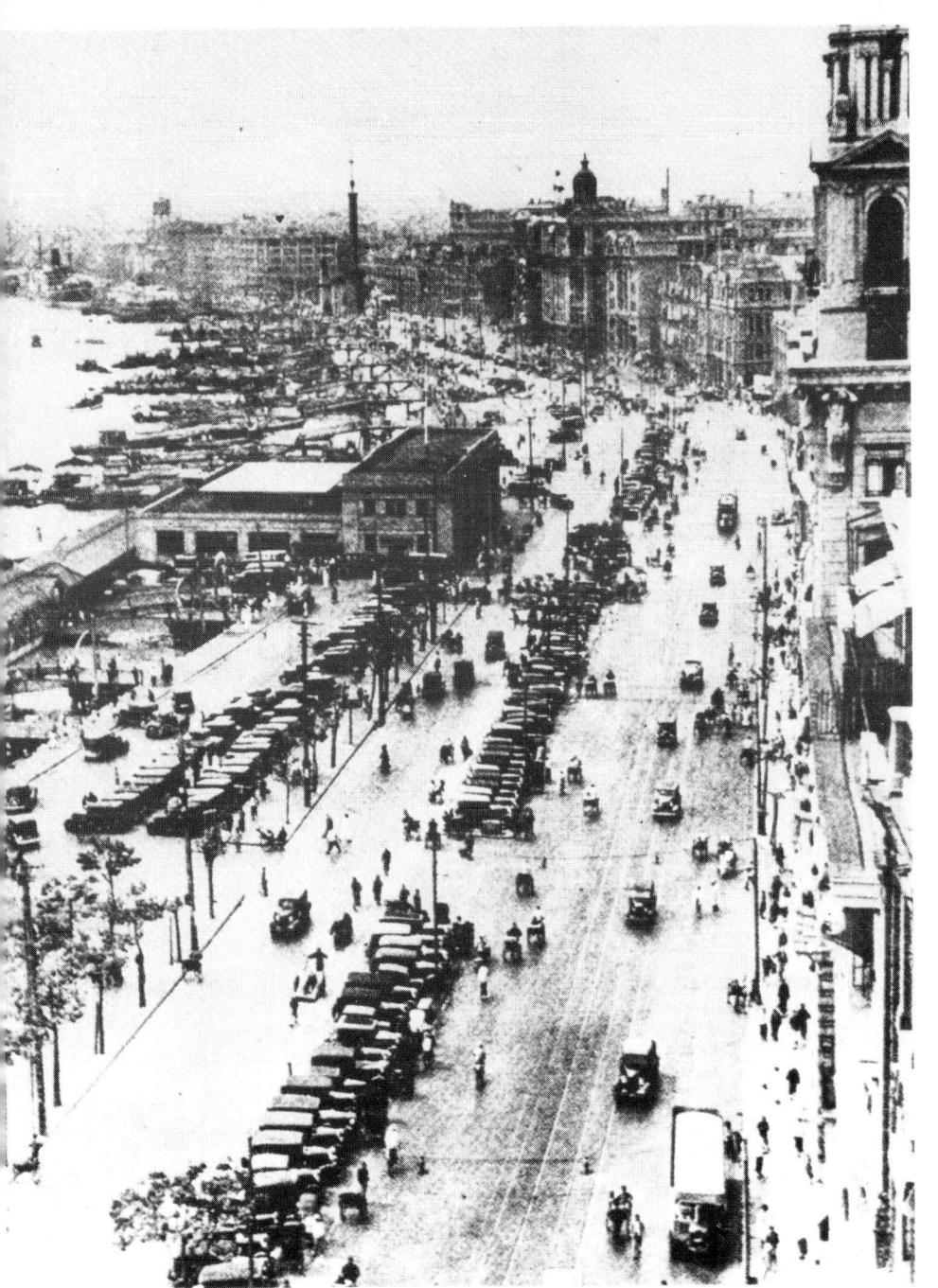

The Bund, Shanghai, in the mid 1930s.

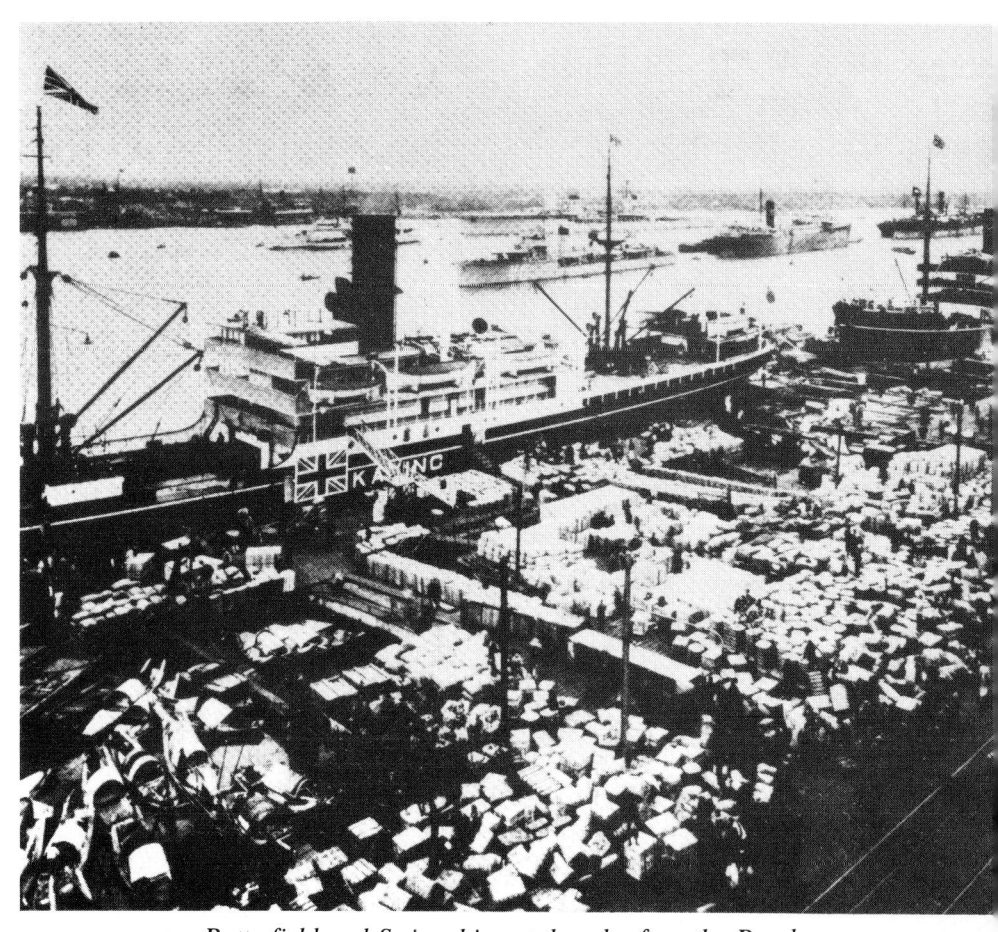

Butterfield and Swire ships at the wharf on the Bund.

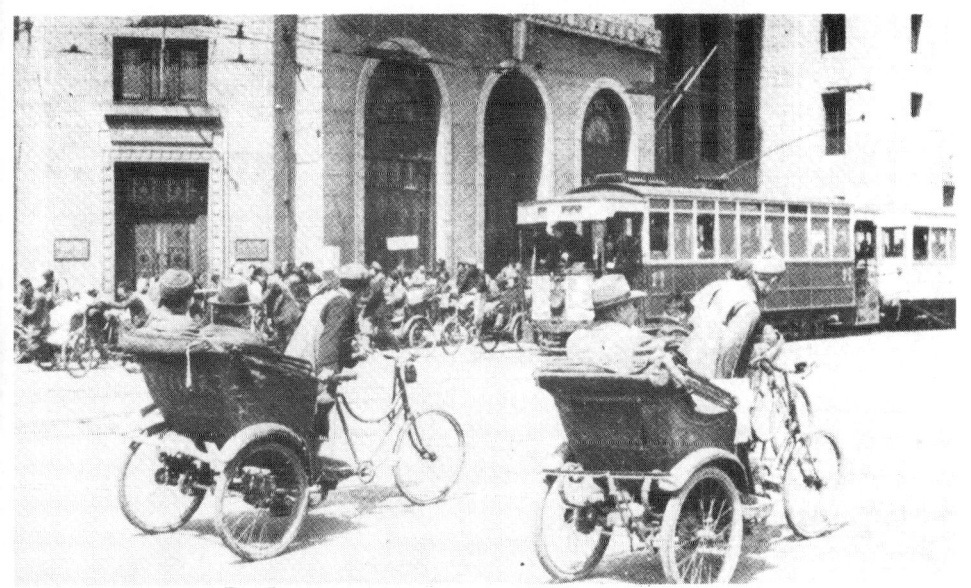

Trishaws were a common mode of transport in Shanghai.

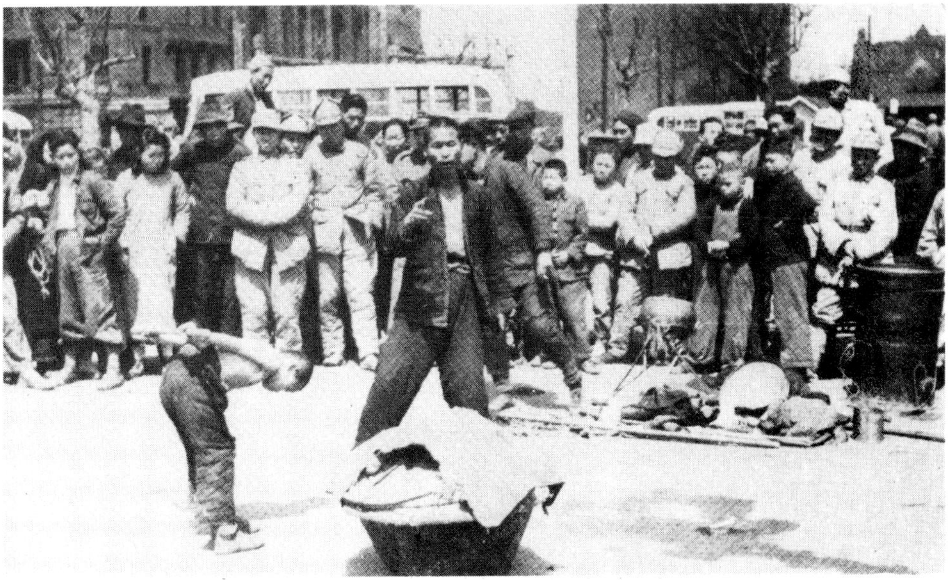

Itinerant acrobats, a frequent sight.

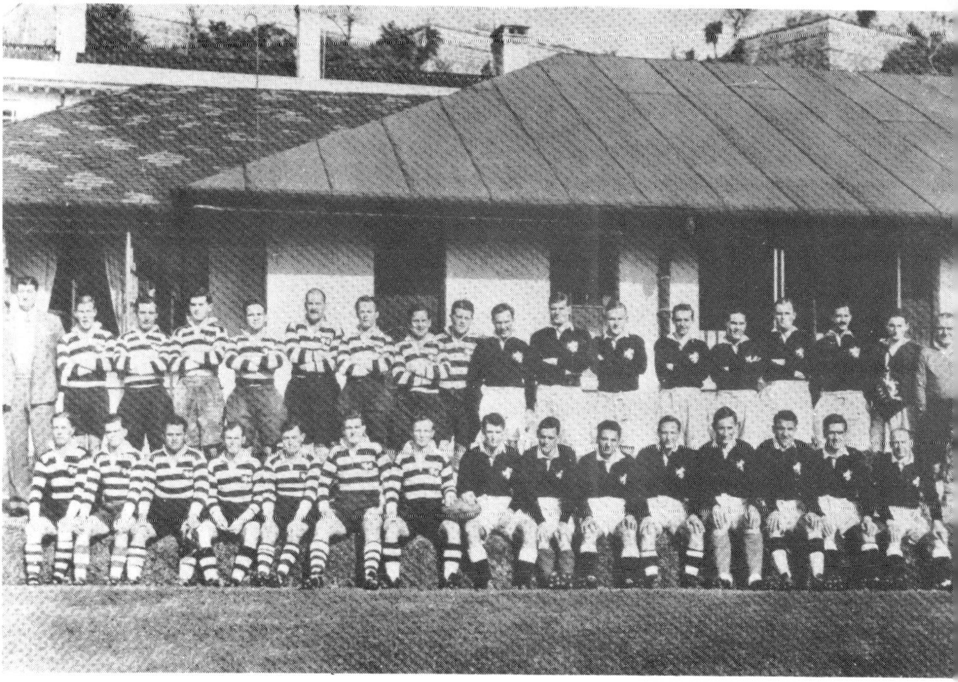

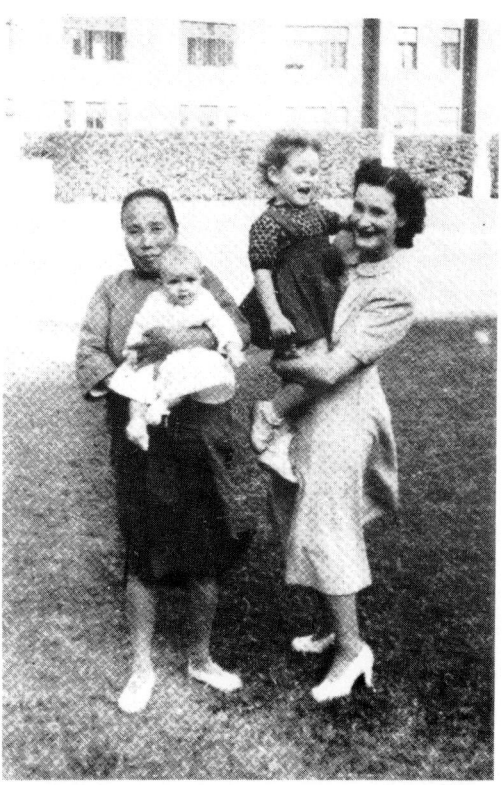

(Above) *The line-up for the last Inter-post match, Hong Kong 1949. Johnnie Henderson was my opposing team-captain.* (Left) *The two girls, Alexi and Corinna, with Jean and the amah Siu Ying* (Little Yellow Bird) *in Shanghai in 1949.*

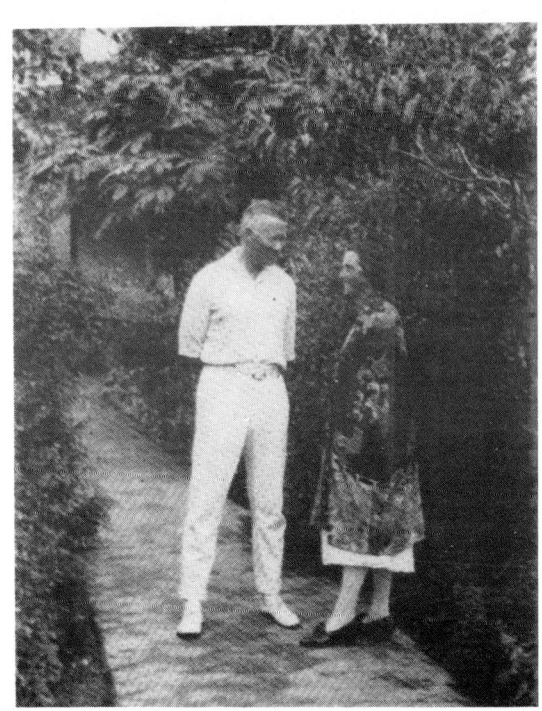

My parents at Chefoo in 1930.

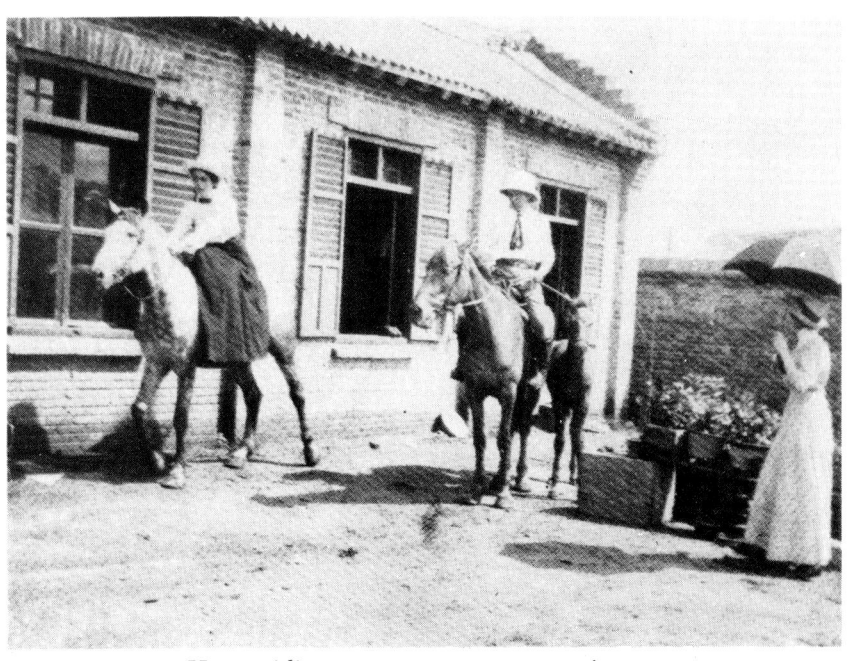

Horse-riding was a common recreation.

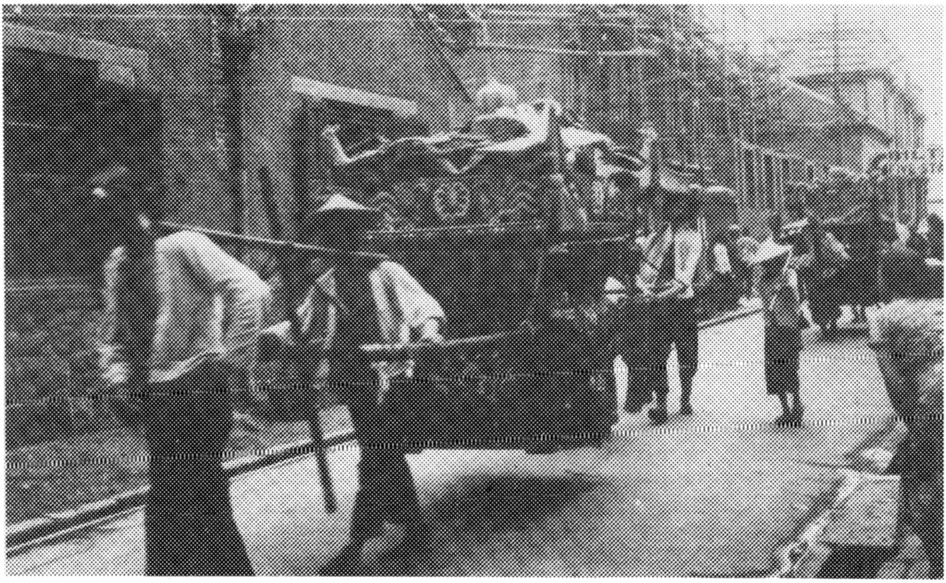

A typical Chinese wedding procession.

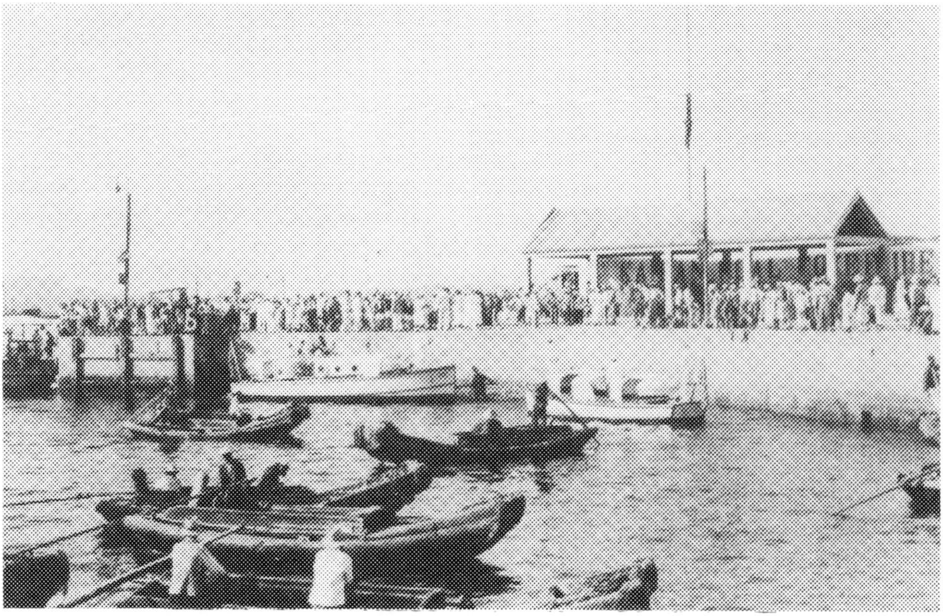

The jetty at Chefoo.

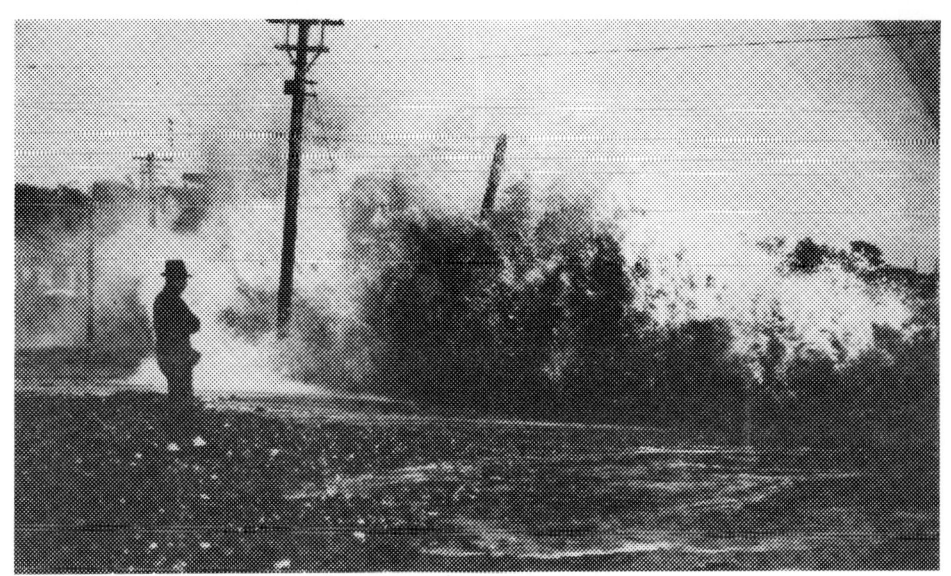

At the height of a storm, Chefoo 1934.

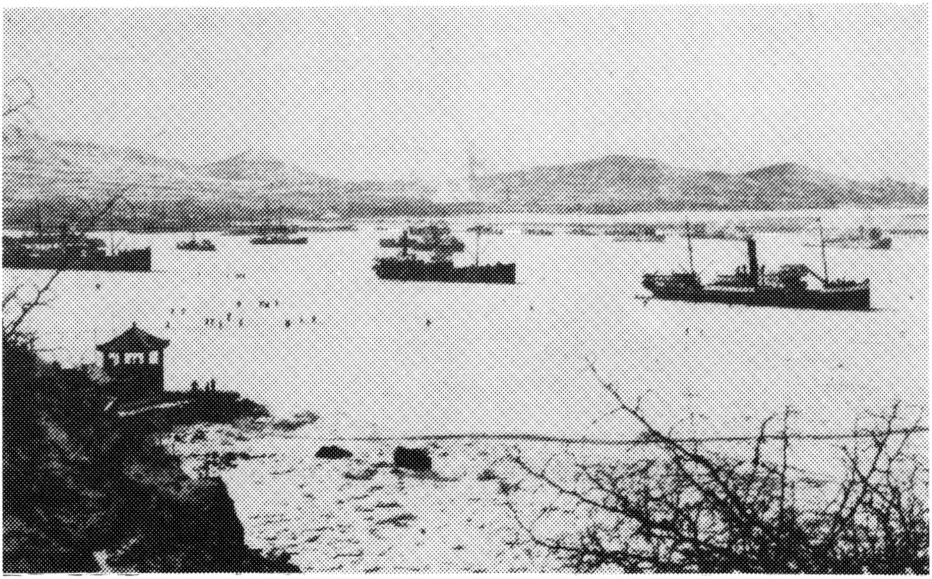

Several ships were frozen into the harbour at Chefoo during the 'Great Freeze' of 1934.

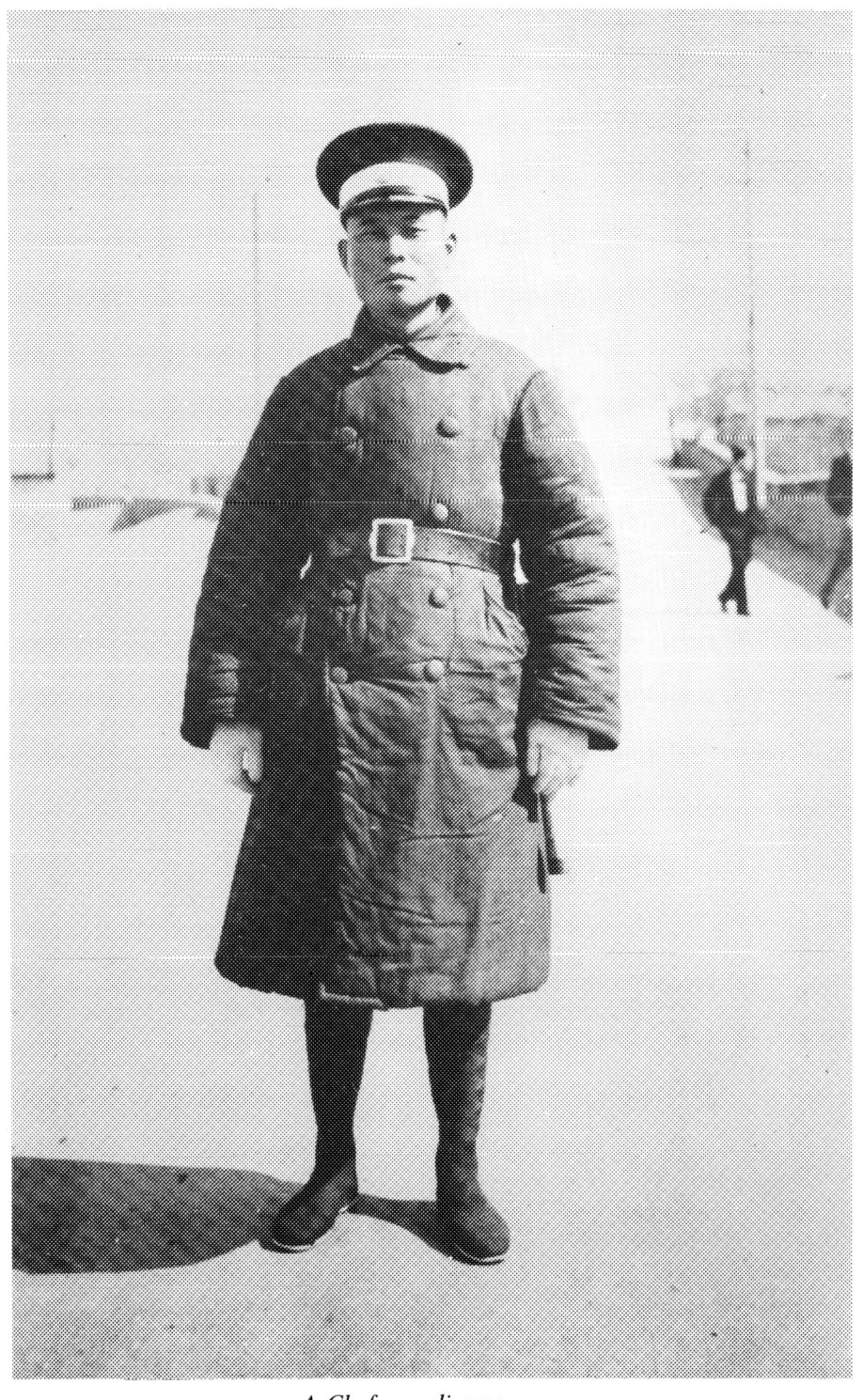

A Chefoo policeman.

Chapter 14

A JOB IN JAPAN

A most difficult letter to write — Jardines help with a loan — Informality in a Japanese train — A house and a car with a story.

Before leaving Shanghai, I had made plans for the future. Our stay in Hong Kong was to be no more than a sojourn. Until late 1950, all foreign and American civilians in Japan had the right to US Army clinics and hospitals. When these facilites were withdrawn, the American and British Chambers of Commerce were faced with yet another problem. They had already been told that shopping on American bases would be reserved only for their army, that army schools would no longer accept the children of civilians, and so on. The two Chambers agreed to sponsor some doctors to set up a clinic. News of this filtered through to Shanghai, as many businessmen, bankers, oil company executives and trading firms looked to Japan from Shanghai and started the tortuous process of getting permission from SCAP. Although SCAP stood for Supreme Commander of Allied Powers, that is General MacArthur, in practice the term included the whole organisation of Government and Occupation; but there was precious little that the eagle eye of the Supremo did not see. I am sure that he knew of the selection of Dr Tom Gentry to set up the clinic.

I was attracted by the possibilities of working in Japan and approached the Manager in Shanghai of the Hong Kong and Shanghai Banking Corporation, to give it the full title, to forward my name to his counterpart in Tokyo and bring it to the notice of the Chambers of Commerce. I told the Manager, George Stacey, that they would need a surgeon and that I had to make plans for my future.

The Hong Kong Bank is one of the great success stories of banking over the last century. They had many branches in China, and the bank's buildings were often the largest and best buildings in the former Treaty ports scattered throughout China, from Manchuria in the north to Canton in the south. They were all written down to one Hong Kong dollar each in the books, so when they were given up to the Communists the profit and loss variation was virtually nil.

The purchaser of one single share of bank stock just before World War I — and people bought single shares in those days — would have had 150 shares in 1973. The purchaser would not have been asked to contribute one extra cent; free issues of shares piled on free issues account for the total. In 1973 it was too expensive to give even one share to your grandchild. They split, ten for one, to bring them to a reasonable figure, so the orginal purchaser had 1,500 of the lesser value. In 1914 there were 80,000 shares; now there are 280 million. Not at all bad considering that the Bank was almost out of business altogether from 1941 to 1945 when Japan occupied all the territories where the Hong Kong & Shanghai Bank traded and had their offices.

Stacey was, in effect, the man next to the Chairman in the Hong Kong head office of the Bank. He was one of the *taipans* in Shanghai, one of the top three or four British businessmen. When I asked for an audience with the great man in his office, he gave me half an hour, listened to my story, and asked me what I wanted. "Would you be kind enough, sir," I asked, "to write a letter on my behalf to the Manager in Tokyo which he can show to the Chamber of Commerce?"

Write the letter yourself," he said. "Mention all your good points. Don't be modest, but try and be truthful. If I agree with it I shall write it as my own letter on official Bank paper and sign it. Have a whisky-soda with me now."

I was overwhelmed, being very small fry in the Shanghai world. I tried to tell him so, especially as I banked — for what my account was worth — with the Chartered Bank. He smiled and laid a hand on my shoulder as he saw me to the door.

It was the hardest letter to compose that I have ever written. It is not difficult to write a letter saying what a wonderful chap you are, how brilliant you are as a surgeon; how you are realiable, honest, humorous and a paragon of all virtues. But it is damn difficult when it is to be signed as though written by a man who is experienced and shrewd, a leading man in his profession and reckoned to be a martinet by his staff. With some fear and trembling the Epistle to the Corinthians was handed to his secretary; Stacey did not alter a word, got it typed out and signed it, and sent me a copy. The note with the copy read, "I have sent it off as it stands with no covering letter of my own. Best of luck." I lost the copy on leaving Shanghai. It would be interesting to know what I thought of myself thirty years ago — I would probably be appalled.

Not banking with the Hong Kong Bank has plagued me ever since.

Later, Stacey himself took over as overall Manager in Japan. He was always kind and we shared the tragedy of his wife's long last illness. He went from Japan to become Deputy Chairman in Hong Kong. Two other close friends have become Deputy Manager over three banking generations. One of them, Martin Curran, was apt to say, "Here he is, staying in our weekend bungalow, not even a member of our congregation although he lives in our parish!"

A few months later I was on my way to Japan. On a September morning the beat of the diesel engine of a Japanese fishing boat sounded through a porthole of the Indo-China Navigation Company's passenger vessel, the *Wing Sang*. Looking out I saw the narrow vessel and her helmsman standing in the stern as she butted her way through the waves sending plumes of spray over her length. The wind was buffeting the wavetops and low clouds and mist were scudding past. Visibility was down to a quarter of a mile. The *Wing Sang* was an hour out of Kobe, soon expecting to make her landfall.

There was little bustle amongst the passengers. Some were on the round trip from Hong Kong and others destined to disembark at Yokohama, but for most of them this was to be their first glimpse of Japan. They lined the rail as the ship nosed her way into port. Apart from a line of hills to the rear, there is little to distinguish Kobe harbour from many others.

The *Wing Sang* was expected to weigh anchor for Yokohama the next day, but Kobe harbour was full of ships, as the Korean War was only three months old. We were to stay there for four or five days and make an additional call at Nagoya. I did not have enough money to pay the train fares and sleeper berths to Tokyo for my wife, two daughters and myself. However, when you have been in the East for long you do not worry. What little capital the Communists had left me on leaving Shanghai in June had been used for our ship's fares and the costs of moving. I went ashore to the Jardine Matheson's office to see the local *taipan*, Robin White. Jardines, the largest trading firm in China, started by Dr Jardine and Mr Matheson during the opium wars, was the greatest of the Chinese *hongs*, as trading firms were called in China. It is still known as the "Princely Hong" and its Kobe representative would hardly refuse to help a passenger on a Jardine ship, travelling at staff rates and under the sponsorship of the British Chamber of Commerce of Japan, of which Jardines were leading lights. Robin sent out for the tickets, telephoned his wife to look after my family, took me out to lunch and gave me 20,000 yen.

"It is an unauthorised expense, Gren. Try to pay it back through the Tokyo office in the next six months!" he said.

As the Americans were the occupying power in Japan, but the Japanese were in local control of the dock, getting our luggage and the wordly goods we had salvaged from China out of the dock was an exercise in the circumvention of bureaucracy. Eventually a US Army sergeant took it upon himself to cut right through the red tape, and with a flourish of his pen he signed across a sheaf of documents. Relieved of responsibility, the Japanese were only too anxious to help, so a small convoy of motor bicycle three-wheelers, with the motor bicycle in front and a cargo platform between the two rear wheels, was loaded with the gear and we set off for the railway station. These three-wheeler transports were legion in the cities and a law unto themselves, weaving in and out of traffic, shuddering to a stop at traffic lights, doing U-turns without warning, and cutting across lines of cars. They shared with the Tokyo taxis the title of "Kamikaze drivers". We only had occasion to use them once again, when our house in Tokyo burned down and they shifted the second instalment of the remnants of our worldly goods. They have been superseded by the march of progress.

The sleeping cars on Japanese trains in 1950 were a fine introduction to one aspect of Japanese life. Berths lined the sides of the carriage and each berth boasted a small curtain which kept the lights from shining directly into one's eyes, but provided the minimum of privacy. The Japanese are not modest about undressing and on departure the passengers were down to their longjohns in no time, parading up and down the aisle, stopping to chat with their neighbours and not a little curious of the foreigners on a civil train. The Americans had their own trains which, incidentally, moved much faster and were a lot more comfortable. There were few foreigners who were both not Americans and without access to the military trains.

We arrived in Tokyo and were met by John Besford, a British dentist. We did not realise how lucky we were that he had received our telegram late at night. Looking back on it, this was a minor miracle, as telegrams could take a week. John had made a trip to

Japan a year previously to scout out the land, and got back into Shanghai on the last day that planes were permitted to land before the Communists took the city. It was imperative for him to get back as his wife and daughter were in Shanghai and, as it happened, no one could leave for six months after the take-over. It was John who first put into my mind the thought of going to Japan.

John Besford took us to have breakfast with the chief of the American International Underwriters in his capacity as Chairman of the American Chamber of Commerce Medical Sub-Committee. He put us in a car and took us to River House which stood by the banks of the Tama River, or Tamagawa, as it is known in Japan. Our gear had already arrived by truck and in our car was a goodly supply of groceries, including a variety of liquor.

"My driver will deliver a car for you tomorrow. It is second-hand but good. You can pay for it after you have started to get going in the clinic," he said as he prepared to leave. He handed me 30,000 yen "to tide you over" and was gone. It seemed to be my day.

The River House had been the Philippine Airlines' staff house. It contained ten bedrooms, all furnished. Only a year later, long after we had left it, did we find out that someone had been murdered in the house and that the airline had moved out. We never saw any ghosts. The car was delivered on time the following day. A year later on selling it, a garage told me that it was obvious from looking at the frame that it had been in a very bad accident, but we never had any trouble with the car; it ran beautifully. As neither my wife Jean nor I are superstitious, we received these two snippets of information with mild interest and no alarm. Perhaps it was better that we did not know about the murder.

Chapter 15

A SURPRISE DEPARTURE

My partnership with Tom Gentry — The Japanese medical examinations — Some dermatological diagnosis — Enter Eugette — A man called E.J. — The limitations of Japanese medicine — The non-existent account books — A partnership ends, another begins.

Tom Gentry was an American with an interesting history which was closely linked with General Claire Chennault. The General had started as a one-man airforce, a soldier — or rather an airman — of fortune. From 1938, flying his Curtis Hawk fighter, he had single-handedly attacked formations of Japanese aircraft as they bombed cities along the Yangtze Valley. Chennault became the friend and confidant of Chiang Kai-shek and his loyalty to Chiang never wavered. He sided with Chiang and became the bitter enemy of "Vinegar" Joe Stilwell who took over the Chinese and American Armies in the Burma-China Theatre when America entered World War II. Stilwell came to hate Chiang Kai-shek and Chennault. In late 1940, the Americans formed the American Volunteer Group or AVG which later became known as the Flying Tigers. The P40 fighters they flew had an air intake just below the propeller hub, on the sides of which were painted the teeth of a tiger.

The Flying Tigers were an airman's or any commander's dream. They were an independent autonomous force, backed up and supplied by the American government, and their purpose was to fight the Japanese Air Force when and where they saw fit. There have been few such forces in history; maybe the parallel was last achieved when Queen Elizabeth I gave her freebooter sea captains a small fleet and carte blanche to ravish the Spanish Main.

The Flying Tigers went into action in favourable circumstances. They moved airfields, and retreated or advanced in their own best interests. This is not to belittle them, for an independent force was strategically the obvious choice. Several of them were very anti-British; they had been taught from childhood that colonialism was wrong and they watched with indifference as the British fought the long Burma retreat and the RAF hurled themselves into oblivion over Rangoon. Relations, however, were not all that bad, as Chiang

Kai-shek paid a Flying Tiger pilot US$500 for every confirmed Japanese aircraft shot down. An RAF pilot would inform an American of the aircraft which he had shot down and on confirmation the US$500 was split.

Tom Gentry volunteered from the US Army as the AVG Medical Officer and set up his medical arrangements in Rangoon in 1940, a year before America entered the war. He stayed with them from their first day until they were amalgamated with the growing strength of the US Air Force in 1942, when Chennault was promoted to Commander of the 14th US Air Force. Tom Gentry became the senior Medical Officer; Chennault stuck by his friends. After the war Chennault formed Civil Air Transport, a quasi-military airline in China which flew anything: people, guns, rice, cargo, warlords, gold, soldiers. As the Communists closed in on city after city, a CAT plane was always the last plane out, crammed with refugees. Tons of rice and supplies were dropped on beleaguered garrisons. CAT gradually became more military and less civil. It eventually retreated to Taiwan to resume its civilian role as the Taiwanese Airline. Chennault, worn out by years of fighting, was getting old and deaf, and the airline shrank in size. Tom Gentry reluctantly looked for new fields and the Tokyo Medical and Surgical Clinic fell into his lap and eventually mine.

This grandiose title covered Tom and me. Suikoshi, 13-1-Chome, Minato-ku was our home. In the manner which sent all foreigners mad, the Suikosha building was the thirteenth building erected in 1 Chome. A Chome, pronounced Cho-May, is a subdivision of a ward of the city and the first house built on it is No. 1; alongside it may be house No. 2356, flanked on the other side by 928 — all very interesting if you want to know how old your residence is, but infuriating if you want to find a specific house; the streets have no names. All this is perfectly logical to the Japanese. Take the train to the nearest station, ask for the local police box and enquire. The local policeman knows everyone in his precinct and is quite likely to walk with you to show the way. While eminently sensible to a Japanese, it reduces the foreigner to tears of vexation, even in the unlikely event of being able to ask for the police box.

Although we had dined together two months previously in Hong Kong, and he had received my letter giving my arrival date, Tom at first did not recognise me and looked slightly baffled when I walked into his office. This deflated my ego, as I had imagined Tom and the community at large were waiting with eager anticipation for his colleague. If anything, he seemed a little put out. But he quickly recovered himself and turned on the charm. When he wanted he could be the most charming of people, making you feel the most awful heel for having harboured any criticism, much less any ill feeling. It was very awkward having to share his office when we had patients simultaneously. This was a temporary situation while the clinic was being constructed next door. Tom was a good organiser and his plans were excellent. The offices were spacious, and looked out on the garden. There was to be an X-ray and darkroom, furniture for the waiting room, equipment for the secretaries, an ample supply of drugs and instruments; we were all ready to go when we had passed the Japanese Medical examination and received our licences to practice. The Chamber of Commerce had lent us the money and was supporting our living until we started practice, had paid the rent for the clinic and of River House and had purchased my car, so I was in debt up to my neck, not forgetting Robin White's 20,000 yen which by then had paled into insignificance. Such is the resilience of a young man that these thoughts caused me no worry whatsoever.

They should have done.

What did worry us was the Japanese medical examinations, and here our worries were unfounded. Having been given the right of entry to Japan by SCAP and thus, by inference, by MacArthur, the Japanese were unlikely to fail us, but we did not realise this at the time. The qualifying examination covered the whole of a student's career from Anatomy and Zoology, basic pre-med subjects, through Pharmacology, Forensic Medicine, Ophthalmology, Ear, Nose and Throat, to Medicine, Surgery and Obstetrics. We sent off for a lot of books but there was no time to study what might be termed "in depth". The Americans publish, or did then, a series of synopses of each subject — A Synopsis of Forensic Medicine, A Synopsis of Pharmacology, etc.; in Britain a similar group was called The Aid to Pathology, The Aid to Biochemistry and so on. They were the sort of books that the unprepared student read through with haste and growing trepidation in the last hour before an examination. The more thorough student affected to despise them. Tom Gentry and I had no option but to order the lot by airfreight.

It was while perusing these once only (there was no time for further study) that one felt the earthquakes. Sitting in an armchair in quiet isolation one would feel a movement, although very slight, at least once every day. While working or in conversation, driving in a car or being active, one would only be aware of a tremor once a month or so, and a major shake every six months. One never got used to the major shakes. The few foreigners who had been through the 1922 Yokohama devastation always ran for an exit, but others sat still. The feeling of helplessness is all-consuming. Back in Edinburgh, while visiting the Professor's Surgical Unit, one of the surgeons asked me if there had ever been an earthquake while I was operating.

"Yes," I said, "and if I had not held onto the patient's right kidney I would have fallen over." A little exaggeration does no harm.

We did pass the Japanese medical examination. My average overall mark was 94 per cent and, taking into account my score in Dermatology of only 5 per cent, this was a brilliant effort, giving me an MD Tokyo. As a student my aim was usually a pass mark, and I do not suppose I ever achieved more than 75 per cent in any exam. My performance in Japan must be attributable either to a new-found genius or that of the Supreme Commander. My licence still holds good. In case any aspiring youngster thinks he can emulate, he had better forget it. We sat and wrote in English by special dispensation. Since the Peace Treaty in 1952 papers have had to be written in Japanese.

The cause of my downfall in Dermatology was my total ignorance of the classification of the forms of fungus which are parasitic on the human body. Ringworm and athletes foot are two well-known manifestations and this was about the extent of my knowledge. Nowadays, when more and more is known about less and less, it is obvious that well-meaning researchers will have evolved a complicated pattern of classification, but for my money it was then, and still is, just plain fungus. However, the passage of time has not robbed me completely of some veritable dermatological diagnostic triumphs.

In 1943 I was in the Air Force as Medical Officer to 353 RAF Transport Squadron based at Palam near Delhi. Palam is now the Delhi International Airport. The station Medical Officer was Flight Lieutenant Ashley. As he was one of the laziest of men, his primary hobby — weight lifting — was out of character. Weight lifting, hypnosis and skin diseases, in that order, were his interests. As the weight lifting club met at six in the evening and hypnosis worked better on a patient after a heavy lunch, the mornings were left free for skin diseases. Because of the comparative infrequency of new cases, Ashley succeeded in stifling his dermatological enthusiasms to such an extent that on many mornings he did not get out of bed early enough to do his sick parade; he left me to do it for him. As there was not much to do at Palam in the mornings, nor for that matter in the afternoons, this suited me fairly well. As he was the acknowledged expert in skin troubles, it was my custom merely to order more of the same treatment. However, one Indian enrolled follower, a sort of uniformed servant or general coolie, had been appearing for many weeks with a rash on his arm. Ashley had gone through the gamut of popular remedies. He had tried a two per cent solution of gentian violet and Unguentum Hydrag Dil, an ointment of dilute ammoniated mercury. He had applied what to me were more exotic remedies — Lassar's paste and his own mixture of calomine lotion with acraflavine. He had even given it a go with hypnosis. Tired of repeating these, and being ignorant of hypnosis, I decided to send the patient to the skin specialist at the nearby Indian Military Hospital, duly filling in Form 41 at some length in order to avoid being advised to use a preparation that had already proved ineffective. An hour or so later I saw the man standing outside the sick quarters waving the Form 41 vaguely in my direction.

"Jaldi Jau IMH," I sternly commanded him. Roughly translated from Hindi this means "Get a move on to the IMH." He still waved the Form 41 in my direction. The fool was waving it at me with the blank side uppermost, and in exasperation I snatched the form and was about to turn it over when something caught my eye. Written on the reverse, right across the page in capital letters, was one word — LEPROSY.

Once in Tokyo and again in Hong Kong about fifteen years later, a similar rash presented itself. I would ask in my letter to the skin specialist if this were leprosy and both times I was right; my acumen rather astounded the skin specialists who took me for a man of broad interests and recondite knowledge.

The results of the exams coincided with the partitioning and completion of the installations in the clinic. At this time Tom intimated to me that his French nurse, Eugette, was coming.

Eugette was not, unless my judgement was in error, pure French. She was either a half or a quarter Vietnamese. French women have always been considered the epitome of femininity and in the East the South Vietnamese women have been acclaimed as the most attractive in Asia. In happier times the Vietnamese wore a long white gown split to the hips at the sides and long black trousers under the gown. This type of dress suited their lithe and graceful figures and movement. Eugette was not lithe, but was very well proportioned indeed; she moved with grace and had the beauty of the Vietnamese superimposed on her French figure; she was very adequate both fore and aft.

When Eugette sailed past a group of men there were no wolf whistles. Instead, simultaneous gasps of incredulity would rob them of breath. I never saw Eugette do any nursing but caught her once cleaning part of our floor by moving a cloth across a smudge in a delicate manner with the toe of a well shod foot. It would have suited me if Eugette had pitched in, so to speak, in a nursing or secretarial role, but these activities she reserved for Tom. She did keep some of his records, mainly copies of the airline pilots' physical examinations. This was useful for Tom, because it saved him from repeating a lot of unnecessary investigations every six months. Later on, Eugette was supposed to keep the accounts.

When the clinic was officially opened we were soon hard at work. One of the first major cases which came my way had many interesting, varied, and important effects on our life in Japan. It was a cold February afternoon when an American came into my office and explained the predicament of E.J.

E.J., as he was known to everyone, was the founder of a trading firm set up in post-war Japan. He had been a close friend of President Roosevelt. The association with the former President was no doubt influential in his being able to set up one of the first trading firms in Japan. We went to the hospital where E.J. was a patient. The doctor there was vainly trying to pass an instrument into the bladder and, as the soft rubber catheter would not pass, he had inserted a metal prong down its length and was using considerable force. There was blood everywhere. E.J. was in great pain and in a state of severe surgical shock. I begged the doctor to desist from his efforts and transferred E.J. to Seibo Hospital. On the way I stopped at the US Army Hospital to borrow an anaesthetist. The condition of the patient demanded the skill of a good anaesthetist as much as a surgeon. Dealing with the immediate surgical problem was not too difficult. When the bladder was opened I found that as a result of a previous prostate operation, the exit had been reduced by scar tissue to a size which permitted the passage of a fine probe. To cut away part of the scar tissue and fashion an adequate channel presented no technical hazard. In contrast, the after-treatment was long, arduous and anxious. As the doctor had by force created a false passage between the urethra and rectum, a vicious pelvic and bladder infection had resulted. The false passage took some weeks to heal, and to say that the post-operative period was stormy is putting it mildly. E.J. was about sixty-eight years old and it was some six months before he was anything like normal. He had to be "followed-up" for several years.

His gratitude to me was permanent and took diverse forms. My wife and family stayed at his country home with him and often he gave us the use of that house for ourselves. Located at Hakone National Park, at a height of 3,000 feet, the house looked out over Lake Hakone towards the hills; beyond, the summit of Mount Fujiyama rose to its perfect snowcapped cone. If you drove across the valley and through a tunnel in the hills, the whole of Fuji was laid before you. It is one of the world's greatest sights.

In winter it can be bitterly cold 3,000 feet up at Hakone, but not in E.J.'s house, which had its own hot spring with the water coursing through the central heating. More effort was expended on turning off radiators than on turning them on. The radiators were firmly screwed off before the log fire was lit in the lounge.

The main joy of the house was the bathroom which boasted a sunken bath two feet below floor level with a tiled surround rising one foot from the floor. You did not sit in the bath; you pushed off from one side to the other. There was no tap, for the hot spring water which flowed all the time, night and day, filled the bath and slopped over the sides onto the tiled floor and out through a drain in the corner. The whole business of having a bath was a glorious exercise of sloshing water about. First you entered and peered about in the steam, then you scooped great scoops of water over the sides when it was too hot. Then you turned the cold full on and, when the waterlevel was down by a foot, finally lowered yourself in when the water was cool enough. Every movement caused more water to spill over the edges. A good push from one side to the other resulted in a tidal wave gushing onto the floor, causing the drain to gurgle away merrily. To spend less than half an hour bathing was an insult to the bath.

My daughters, Corinna and Alexi, went wild when they had girls of the same age staying as guests. The sight of half a dozen girls of ages three to seven making a divine mess of spashing was entertainment for the parents. When it was understood that parents were to be allowed to be spectators the girls modestly donned their bathing suits.

E.J. was an influential man, and a month or two before the Peace Treaty was signed, he acted as intermediary between one of the largest American Oil companies and Mitsubishi to build a tanker in Japan. It was the first of many such deals.

To celebrate the contract, E.J. held a cocktail party. The top men were there and in view of the importance of the occasion, Prince and Princess Chichibu attended. E.J. asked me along. A Japanese would never dream of asking his doctor or surgeon to such an affair. The guest list would be carefully made up of the highest grades of industrialists, with perhaps a senior banker and the Minister of Transport. Anyone unconnected with the business would not even be thought of, and as a Prince of the Royal blood was to be present, the list was correspondingly more exclusive.

One of the guests found me in the corner and was surprised to hear my title.

"Ah, you are a doctor of Science or Metallurgy?" he got out with some difficulty.

"No," I replied, "I am a surgeon practising in Tokyo."

He was baffled, and became even more baffled when he found out that I was British and not American.

I then asked him who he was and he produced his card. T.S. Sensui was printed in large letters, and underneath in smaller script was Liquidator in Chief, Mitsubishi Heavy Industries. Down in the left-hand corner in very small print was Chief Liquidator Mitsubishi Heavy Industries.

At this time the Allies were making efforts to disperse the three great *zaibatsu*, or trading firms, of Mitsui, Mitsubishi and Sumitomo. There is no exact equivalent elsewhere to one of the *zaibatsu*. They were so diversified. It would not be impossible to board a Mitsui ship in London built from steel made in Mitsui Steelworks Ltd., constructed at Mitsui Engineering and Shipbuilding Co. Ltd., insured by Taisho Marine and Fire Insurance Co. Ltd. (a Mitsui subsidiary), financed by the Mitsui Bank, fuelled by the General Sekiyu Oil Co. with Mitsui control and so on. When the passenger got off in Yokohama, the chances were that the taxi he stepped into would be a Bluebird — made by Datsun, which was partially owned by Mitsui. Needless to say, General Sekiyu Oil is back again, since they will have filled the tank!

"Mr Sensui," I said. "I expect you are liquidating Mitsubishi Heavy Industries in such a way that they can all be put together again very quickly."

He looked surprised, taken aback. He quickly recovered, guffawed with laughter and said, "You are British, you are quite right."

Two years later, when Japan had become independent and E.J. had negotiated a few more tankers, almost exactly the same party was held. The Prince and Princess were there again, so was Sensui and so was I. Approaching Sensui, I repeated our previous conversation nearly word for word till he remembered me and then he looked even more astounded than the first time. I had not forgotten his name but I wanted to see his card so I professed ignorance. He gave it to me. T.S. Sensui it said in large letters. Underneath was Manager in Chief, Mitsubishi Heavy Industries, and down in the left hand corner in very small print Chief Manager, Mitsubishi Heavy Industries.

On another occasion E.J. was not feeling well and he asked Jean and me to look after his guests; Mr and Mrs Schlitz they may as well be called, because he was president of the Schlitz Beer Company of Milwaukee, and E.J.'s firm had the agency for Japan, Korea and Okinawa. They came to pick us up at our house in E.J.'s chauffeur-driven car; we were to go to Yokohama for a pleasure trip across Tokyo Bay in a launch. The Schlitzes were not at all impressed by anything they had seen in Japan: Tokyo was dilapidated, the traffic suicidal. They had not enjoyed Japanese food, especially an offering of raw fish, which is not at all bad when one gets used to it.

Jean, feeling herself to be in the role of hostess, defended both the place and the people. She remarked that some Americans who had been brought up in Japan and spoke good Japanese became very pro-Japanese as a result of understanding them. There was to be one such in the party and they would enjoy meeting and talking to Bill. The morale of the Schlizes rose when we boarded the launch and they were able to mix with a crowd of fellow compatriots; Bill particularly impressed them. The launch set out across the bay. The water became choppy, and the guests of honour found it advisable to retire to the cabin and lie down until calmer seas were reached under the lee of Chiba Peninsula. The launch anchored alongside some fishing smacks in order to negotiate for some of the catch. One or two rather good-looking fish were purchased by Bill who had boarded the smack and was in deep conversation with the owner. While the Schlitzes, who had reappeared on deck, watched with interest, the fisherman presented Bill with two small fish roughly the size of sardines.

To my surprise and to the horror of our guests, Bill cut off the heads of the fish, suspended one by the tail between fingers and thumb, tilted back his head, poised the fish over his open mouth and dropped it in whereupon it disappeared down his gullet without much sign of swallowing. Instantly the second was dealt with in an exactly similar manner. If that is what happened to Americans who lived in Japan, the Schlitzes wanted no part of it; they retired and lay down again. There was a minimum of conversation on the return trip to Tokyo.

E.J. some time that summer became a member of the Medical Sub-Committee of the Chamber of Commerce. I wrote him a letter about the affairs of the clinic which he filed in case of future need. It turned out to be a very important letter indeed for me.

I visited E.J. and Freddie, his wife, ten years later when he was living down the Peninsula in San Francisco. He was nearly eighty by then and had suffered a stroke from which he had recovered completely, except for one bizarre consequence. He remembered people's names, and all the events of his life, but his memory for place names had been almost obliterated. We spent half a morning together and the conversation went something like this.

"You remember when you came to our house in . . .," he shook his head in irritation, "that place where we both lived."

"Tokyo," I said.

"There you are, you see, Tokyo, but do you know that three minutes from now the name will have escaped me again. It is extremely annoying, sometimes I forget that Washington is the capital and heaven knows we spent enough time there."

Freddie said goodbye to me in the house but E.J. came out to the car. I think he knew that he did not have much more time. He took my hand in both of his. He was tall and distinguished.

"You saved my life in Tokyo," he said. "See, I remember the name, your visit has been good for me. Only this morning before you came, I said to Freddie that in many ways these last ten years have been the best and most rewarding of our lives. You gave me those ten years. Both Freddie and I want to thank you."

He grasped my hand again through the car window.

He died a few months later.

The US Army Hospital in Tokyo was the rear base unit for casualties of the Korean War. That it maintained the facilities for foreign civilians of all nationalities until the end of 1950 was more surprising than the closing of its doors to all except for army and embassy people. Doctors and surgeons of the highest order staffed the hospital. Many times I sought their advice and never failed to get not only aid but patient consideration of my problems and help from their X-ray and laboratory departments. As they were so obviously totally busy for long hours, their co-operation was deeply appreciated. The Chief Surgeon, Colonel Matuska, went out of his way on several occasions. Every surgeon has cases which go wrong and he then desperately needs advice and encouragement; the reassurance of another opinion is in itself of inestimable value.

Japanese medicine at that time was suffering from many deficiencies, but the three main ones stemmed from the following; sketchy education of the students during the war; the stultifying effect of a military dictatorship which had halted all development of original thought, research and progress for over a decade (the standard practice and teaching were based on those of their German ally of 1938 vintage), and lastly, there was a ghastly shortage of material and equipment.

My chief nightmare was anaesthesia. We relied completely on open ether — ether dropped on a mask. A Japanese anaesthetist could only be cajoled into giving a sufficient dose by a combination of patience and encouragement. The amount of ether administered drop by drop which would anaesthetise a slim Japanese of 120 lbs. would hardly begin to affect a robust hard-drinking Dutchman of 200 lbs. The Occidental generally requires much more anaesthetic than an Oriental. If the anaesthetists did finally manage to get the patient under, it became second nature to me to listen to the patient's breathing, to try to anticipate not the giving of too much, but of the patient coming half awake and starting to struggle. It does not help a surgeon continually to have to watch the anaesthetic, to deal with tight instead of relaxed abdominal muscles, to study the colour of the blood in the wound lest it become dark from poor oxygenation, to peek over the screen at intervals to look at the colour of the patient's face, and generally to have a double responsibility.

Suture material was another bugbear. The Japanese used plain sewing thread for all ordinary purposes, and small stitch abscesses were the order of the day. I asked one of the young surgeons at Seibo Hospital if they had much trouble with wound infection. "None, or hardly ever," was his answer.

I soon discovered that by wound infection we meant completely different things. He considered a wound infection to be a riproaring inflammation in which the wound was likely to break open completely and discharge pus by the cupful. Stitch abcesses around the skin sutures were so commonplace as not to be classified as infections at all.

To have a parcel delivered by the Post Office was to try to pass a camel through the eye of a needle. When I made trips to Hong Kong or the United States I bought sufficient silk and catgut suture material to fill up our stocks. There was never any difficulty bringing it through the airport customs in my baggage. Half my luggage consisted of surgical supplies and instruments, and it was well worthwhile having to pay excess baggage charges. I complained gently about this once to a fellow airline passenger. He listened with sympathy and then told me his own problems which put mine into insignificance. He ran a factory of some sort in Nicaragua. To import small parts necessitated bribes, paper work, and a minimum of six months' waiting, frequently ending in the total loss of the items. He made twice yearly trips to Europe and the United States and usually took back over 2,000 lbs. of excess baggage.

"It takes me longer to get through the formalities at the airport but eventually it all comes out with me," he said. "It is costly but it is the only way I can keep my factory going. It is well worth the cost."

If a surgeon in America or Britain were asked how many packets of plain catgut, chromatic catgut, silk or nylon he used in six months it would be surprising if he had the faintest idea. One gets through the material at a fast rate and, more because of the depletion of the supply than a Scottish meanness, I gradually become adept at getting more and more ties out of a given length of suture. When watching surgeons at work since, the profligate way the theatre nurse breaks out a new length of catgut when they have discarded a piece with a couple of good ties left in it never fails to make an impression on me. This habit has stayed with me; some ten years later in Hong Kong the Chinese theatre sister put a new piece of silk in my hand as I was making a tie with a short length. It had become a joke with the theatre staff.

"Try using a new bit, Dr Wedderburn," she said, "but please be careful. We use the money we save with you to pay for our Christmas party."

Another feature of the practice of medicine in Japan which was reprehensible was the reluctance of doctors to get a second opinion. This attitude was not confined to one's own speciality. The Chief Surgeon at Seibo Hospital never approached the physician to give an opinion on a surgical case with concomitant heart disease. The junior in his own unit was expected to assess the dangers and provide treatment. If and when the patient survived the surgical assault he might be handed over for further study and care.

I learned this lesson at an early stage when investigations suggested that a young wife had a tumour of the small intestine. The tumour was in the pelvis, so I asked the gynaecological specialist at the Bluff Hospital in Yokohama to examine her, to exclude a gynaecological lesion. Glancing at the operation list on my next visit, I found that the patient's name had been included on the list for operation by the gynaecologist. This perturbed me and I mentioned it to Dr Morton, who was the Superintendent.

"Don't you know," he said, "that he assumed that you are unwilling to do the case yourself? To ask him to see her is tantamount to handing over the case. He told me that the pelvic examination was normal but that he was quite willing to tackle it."

Morton had to exercise great tact with the doctor before we ended up doing the operation together. He made the incision and I carried on from there.

A similar incident happened much later. Crohn's Disease, Regional Iletis, affects both the end of the small intestine and the beginning of the large intestine. President Eisenhower had the doubtful distinction of being the most illustrious person to harbour the disease. At a surgical meeting, a foreign surgeon had given a lecture on the condition. In the discussion afterwards the Japanese surgeons voiced their interest, but declared that the Japanese do not get Crohn's Disease, so it was interesting for me to operate on a classical case in a Japanese.

I performed a short circuit or bypass, that is to join the gut above and below the affected area and make an opening between the pieces of gut. This allows the gut content to pass through the opening and not through the loop of diseased intestine. Nowadays this procedure is reckoned to be all that is necessary, but in 1952 the diseased segment was excised at a second operation. Thinking that it would be of interest to a Japanese I asked Nakayama, the Chief Surgeon in Seibo Hospital, to see the case, as the patient was a Japanese. A few days later, to my dismay, Nakayama had him on his operating list. After some negotiation, the tactic of both of us operating was adopted again. Nakayama was a nice old boy of over seventy, who would not have dreamed of trying to offend me. He had just come to the same conclusion as the gynaecologist at the Bluff. The sequel was interesting; Nakayama declared that it was tuberculous disease, moderately common in Japan. The area affected by both diseases is the same part of the gut. Seibo Hospital pathological laboratory reported the specimen as tuberculosis; it was diplomatic to do so — Nakayama had said it was. After all, the Japanese do not get Crohn's Disease. However, I had cut out two or three pieces from the specimen and taken them to the US Army Hospital laboratory. I did not use any diplomacy, but told the pathologist the facts and awaited his verdict. He called me up, and said that it was a typical Crohn's.

I said nothing about this at Seibo. A modicum of loss of face, for me, was well worthwhile to keep our relations on a friendly basis.

The return of the Army Hospital to its military functions presented us with a ready-made practice; the Bluff Hospital filled the need in Yokohama. Originally Yokohama was the port for the Kanto area of Japan, but the two cities of Tokyo and Yokohama now form a continuous metropolitan area. River House stood on the Tama River which was the dividing line between the two, I visited Bluff Hospital twice a week. The Superintendent, Dr Milton C. Morton, had been attached to the medical administration of the occupying power. His knowledge of many aspects of medicine in Japan, from auxiliary services such as drug firms to many of its most illustrious doctors, was much wider than mine. He was a useful man to know; he could steer one through the intricacies of bureaucratic procedure when I would have floundered and probably given up the effort.

Our clinic was soon showing very active signs of life. We could forsee our debts being wiped out and could even expect a mild prosperity. Tom Gentry was very much the man who maintained liaison with the American Chamber of Commerce. Indeed, he created an aura of mystique in this regard from which I was excluded. When I needed money he would grudgingly hand me out a packet of yen which made me feel rather like a junior lieutenant receiving a favour from his colonel. Considering that I had reached the exalted rank of

Wing Commander in the RAF, equivalent to a Lt. Colonel, this irked me. Although I did not admit it to Tom, the dizzy height of Wing Commander was temporary, unpaid, and I suspect, a mistake somewhere in headquarters. Nevertheless, there was no question that I had been the equivalent of a major. The fact that no signs of bookkeeping were discernible made me concerned. True, from time to time Tom would be seen jotting down items on pieces of paper about the size of a visiting card, but his jottings were unintelligible to me, especially when viewed upside down from across his desk. After a decent interval of a month or two I tackled him on the subject, only to be told that Eugette was keeping the books. She did this work in their apartment because, he said, it was wiser to move them away from prying eyes for reasons of security and tax, or shall we say tax evasion? For some time I accepted this state of affairs with only minor reservations; most of my energies and interests were directed towards building up the practice and establishing a surgical reputation. We were so obviously in a position to achieve this, and the opportunity was so patently promising that there seemed to be no reason to have any doubts, until one day an incident occurred which stopped me in my tracks.

Tom and Eugette announced that they were leaving for business reasons for America. They would be away for two weeks.

"It would be better," I suggested to Tom, "if Eugette gave me the books to keep while you are away."

"I'll get her to bring them down this afternoon." They did not arrive. On leaving the office in the evening I met Eugette in the corridor. She was dressed up to travel and looked like a million dollars.

"Eugette," I said, "Tom said you would give me the account books before you left."

"What account books?"

It was easy to keep your mind on a figure but not on accounts when you looked at Eugette. She was puzzled for a moment, but if you are as good-looking as Eugette you do not worry your pretty little head with such mundane matters.

"Have a good trip," I said. She turned and flowed down the corridor like a stream of quicksilver. The accounts books quite obviously did not exist.

This revelation marked a turning point in my association with Tom. John Besford, the dentist who shared our office, advised me, after I had put the problem to him, to send out my own accounts and to keep my own records and a very accurate set of records at that. My relations with Tom cooled perceptibly from the time of his return but this method worked fairly well. It is remarkable that no open breach took place; we had lunch together occasionally and the subject of finance was always avoided. Any time there was a lull in the conversation I would ask him about some aspect of the war in China and he would be off on some reminiscence of hurried retreats and evacuations or about the bombing of Chung King.

This uneasy peace could hardly be described as a satisfactory way of conducting our affairs but so it went on for almost a year. Eventually I approached a doctor, Bernard Rosenberg, whom I had known in Shanghai. Bernard and his wife, both in their early forties, had left Berlin for Shanghai a few weeks before Hitler seized power. There they had found the competition fierce and had had several lean years. He had spent some time in Australia before settling in Japan. I did not know Bernard well but we discussed the possibility of my pulling out of the clinic and setting up with him. Bernard had just passed the Japanese qualifying exams, and we were at the stage of trying to formulate our plans. His problems were simple but mine were complex because of my obligations to the American and British Chambers of Commerce, obligations which were both financial and moral. To find a way through the intricacies of the deadlock was no easy task, especially as the Americans quite naturally would place more trust in the word of Tom, a fellow national.

One day, while still groping for a solution, Tom asked me to lunch with him. We chatted away on amiable terms until we had reached the coffee stage.

"By the way," said Tom, "Eugette and I are leaving for the States today."

This did not occasion surprise as he often went off for a few days to Taiwan to see Chennault and had been to the States on one trip already.

"How long do you expect to be away?" I asked.

"We are not coming back!"

There are a host of words and expressions in the English language to describe my feelings. The word of my choice was pole-axed.

"Well," said Tom cheerfully, "Eugette and I are busy; we have a lot of packing and things to clear up." He got to his feet, lunch was over.

"Look here, Tom, you can't just go off like that. What about the American Chamber, all the finance and so on? We must have a talk about it and come to some arrangements," I remonstrated.

"All right," he replied, "I shall see you in the restaurant here at half past five."

I tottered down to the office. Glancing at Onodasan, our secretary, a daughter of Baron Onoda, I realised that she was not our secretary; she was my secretary. Shegasan was my nurse, Sakodasan, the radiographer, was my radiographer, the laboratory technician was mine alone. I reflected on the date, the 28th March, three days to pay day, plus the rent. Turning the combination to open the safe door in some trepidation, I found it to be barren except for some documents. The whole organisation had been planned for at least three doctors, and now there was one.

Somehow I got through the afternoon and went up to the restaurant. By six, Tom had not come down from his room, so I took the lift to the third floor. The door of their room was ajar, the beds were stripped, an empty Kleenex box was on the floor, and other discarded items were littered about. I looked into the bathroom foolishly wondering if they might be there. It was not empty — a maid was cleaning up.

"Where is Dr Gentry?" I asked.

The maid looked surprised. "They left for Haneda Airport at four o'clock."

Suikosha was dry but there was a bar close by. I had withstood the first shock but the second needed first-aid. Two very large Scotch whiskies downed in rapid succession did little to alleviate my distress. When I got home my stricken look was immediately apparent to Jean.

'What has happened?" she asked with concern.

"Get me a drink, dear. Gentry has left for good. What a mess we are in, the whole shooting match is now my responsibility, debts and all."

"Well, not quite, dear, you will have Bernard Rosenberg to help you."

"What do you mean?" I asked. The thought of him had been driven from my mind.

"You must know."

"I must know what?" I asked.

"He was on the phone an hour ago. Don't you know he will be

112

taking Gentry's share?" The Scotch whisky was taking an awful beating.

"Have you his phone number?" I asked.

I think I was a bit incoherent on the telephone but I arranged to go to his house straightaway. In a flash we were in the car, not forgetting the bottle of whisky; as he was German I thought he might have peculiar alcoholic leanings. I need not have worried. Bernard always had a plentiful supply of the right stuff.

In the East I have been associated with some twenty-five partners at one time or another. Some of them are my very good friends, one or two I despise, but Bernard Rosenberg, a German-Jew from Berlin who fought as a private in the German Army in Rumania in World War I (from the photographs he showed me they certainly did not look like a crack unit), was one of the finest men I have ever met and the best partner I have had.

Chapter 16

THE MAN WHO CAME TO DINNER

A housewarming party that ends up with a crash — Paddy and Paul move in and Paul stays — A well-balanced partnership — Squaring up the accounts with the Chamber of Commerce.

A new era opened for the clinic when Bernard Rosenberg joined; we at last set up a proper accounting procedure. As a friend of mine, Duncan Fraser, had just married "Miss BOAC of 1950/51" in Tokyo, her husband, Bernard and I decided that she was ideally qualified for the job. Mary Fraser was not consulted, but just told to turn up for work. Mary has a very strong character and it was only a combination of being pitchforked into life in a small Japanese house in Katase-cho, soon known as "Catastrophecho" together with the charisma of early marriage, that permitted this high-handed dictatorial attitude to meet with success. The accounts system was born and grew up with Mary. To be elected Miss BOAC was a tribute not only to her good looks but also to her character and personality. Delinquents in the matter of payments were greeted with charm or withering contempt as best fitted the occasion; she produced results. We sought some professional advice at the beginning but thereafter the accounts were not only created but kept immaculate.

As Duncan was at that time a member of the lower orders in his firm, he was furnished with housing, but the house was not of a high standard. It had two floors with a rickety stair and had no pretensions of being called semi-western style. It was frankly pure Japanese and jerry-built at that; to lean against a wall was to invite disaster. Hardly had they moved in before Duncan cut his hand badly when a porcelain tap (faucet) broke as he was turning it off one Sunday morning. He appeared at my house, and I took him into the kitchen for repairs as blood was dropping all over the place. My eldest daughter rushed next door to summon a host of our neighbour's children with the remark: "Come quickly, there is a man bleeding in our house."

My daughters and the six Ryan girls formed a tight circle of spectators as I got out the local anaesthetic and suturing material. It was the best Sunday morning entertainment they had enjoyed for many months.

When Duncan recovered from his injury he decided to hold a housewarming party. A conspicuous guest was Dick Partridge, the house's previous occupant who, as the party got going, tried to dissuade Dr Becker, a German lawyer, from feeding olives to the tropical fish. The fish tank was still being housed by the Frasers until Dick was settled in his new house and Dr Becker, a frequent visitor, had in the past indulged in this habit which resulted in a huge mortality amongst the sword-tails, neon tetras and other exotic members of the fish population.

The room, converted from its bare Japanese design to the semblance of a lounge, was designed for one or two soft-footed Japanese. The builder had not visualised some twenty hefty foreigners with their wives and girlfriends jumping about with glasses filled to the brim. The party hotted up and Dr Becker decided to give the fish their quota of olives. Dick tried to restrain him but Becker started to throw the olives across the room. At this point a warning groan from the floor made everyone stop and as an olive floated across the room the whole floor gave way with an alarming crash to land on the solid earth of Japan some three feet below. Down went the surprised guests, the hosts, chairs, ornaments and drinks. The fish tank leaned over at an angle and stayed poised temporarily for a few seconds. Dick thrust towards it to save his few remaining pets but just as he got into position to reach up to the tank, now above him, more of the floor subsided and Dick received most of the contents — but not all. Two girls just picking themselves up got the remainder. A sword-tail disappeared into the bra of one of them where it proceeded to wriggle with gusto. This sword-tail was born doubly lucky; it was retrieved and put in a glass of water, the sole survivor of the holocaust. The party continued unabated at a lower level. Becker maintained that his last olive shot plopped into the tank, a direct hit, but no guest could corroborate the claim.

Unsure of legal responsibility under Japanese law for this mishap, Duncan and Dick decided to make their own repairs next morning. Somewhat the worse for wear, they viewed the lounge where a hole, open from below to all the winds that blew, faced them instead of a floor. Going to a neighbouring garage they borrowed a hydraulic jack and, by dint of raising the floor at the centre and shoring it up with a few pyramids of bricks, they had it back in position, more or less, by lunchtime. True, the floor creaked and groaned, sagged and wavered, and cracks and splinters marred its symmetry, but they purchased an incredibly cheap piece of carpet for 2,000 yen which they spread over the floor and hammered down with tacks. There was always a feeling of insecurity and a certain spice of danger crossing the Frasers' lounge thereafter, but the floor held firm and no further repairs were, as far as we know, ever necessary. It may be there to this day.

Right opposite the Frasers' house was a building called the Fuji Hotel with a large flashing sign advertising the Japanese baths available inside. When conversation flagged it was interesting to watch the GIs and their Japanese girlfriends checking in; they certainly seemed to need a great deal of washing and bathing. I told Mary that this establishment raised the whole tone of the area.

Not for nothing was their house called "Catastrophecho".

It was about this time that Jean decided she should make a trip home to Scotland with Corinna and Alexi. We had been three years in Shanghai and eighteen months in Tokyo; there seemed little possibility of my taking leave for a long time. In fact, over six years were to pass between the time I left for China and my first visit back to the United Kingdom. Not wanting to live alone in a rambling house, I searched around for a companion and found Paddy Ryan of the Hong Kong Bank. He suggested that another Irishman, Paul Donnelly, be added to our number. When Jean and the girls went off from Yokohama, the two Irishmen moved in. Paddy and Paul were both Catholics and both small men; I suppose Paddy was about 5'5", but Paul stood a diminutive 5'2". Paul had rather a red complexion, a receding hairline and skin drawn tightly over the bones of his face and forehead. He also had an amazing capacity for Scotch whisky. When out at a party he must have taken in an amount pound for pound which would put a large six-foot man on his back. When everyone else was willing to call it a day Paul would insist on another round. Anyone who refused was called a "piker". I do not know a single one of his friends who was not given this label, and he could put a wealth of contempt and disgust into two simple words — *"You piker."*

I don't know if "piker" is an Irish term, but when delivered by Paul there was never any doubt as to what it meant. On the occasions when we all dined together they argued hammer and tongs about Irish politics and the relations with England, leaving England very much with the short end of the stick. The turbulent years of Anglo-Irish differences were laid at the door of the English although the Scots were not blameless, more to be pitied than held responsible. I would sit back and let them argue; to have expressed an opinion would have banished their Irish differences and made them stand together to vent Celtic wrath on my head.

Paul became my good friend and later a good friend of my family. His knowledge of the bars, even in the quiet suburb in which we lived, was monumental. There was no time of day or night that Paul could not find a small place open down the quietest street with hardly more than a bench, a table, a bar and one barmaid in attendance. The barmaids everywhere knew him as Bingsan, owing to some peculiar Japanese view that he bore a strong resemblance to Bing Crosby.

He was popular with the girls but a bit offhand. He chased the singer in the Casablanca Dance Hall off and on for a couple of years, but the courtship progressed slowly because the only time he ever got to the Casablanca, a large cheap dance hall forming the roof of Shibuya Railway Station, was when we or he alone left Yokohama and we passed Shibuya on our way home.

We would rush up the stairs at about ten minutes to one to catch the singer in her rendering of the last number of the evening, a Japanese translation of "Goodnight Sweetheart". Paul would station himself in front of the grandstand and start making advances as the roll of drums announced that the evening's music was finished; by then the supply of beer had been stopped so he could not even give his ladylove a drink. Maybe she lived in hope that some day Bingsan would drop in around midnight. The last part of the last dance courtship seemed an unsatisfactory way of conducting a love affair. The only medal Paul got from this, in my estimation and in the singer's, was one for persistence. I do not think he ever made much progress.

A couple of pals of Paul's came to Japan for a week and were immediately invited to stay. One of them, the Honorary Irish Consul in Hong Kong, Dermot Nolan, told me that he was a bit mystified at the way in which I used to turn up, have a meal and a drink and disappear to bed with the word "piker" ringing in my ears. It was not till many years later when we met again that he realised that it was my house and not Paul's. Not that Paul was like that; he was completely without pretension, and had just not bothered to explain the matter.

NO LOTUS GARDEN

When Jean and the girls returned from Scotland, Paul was supposed to start looking for somewhere to live. A week and then a month went by. When we moved from the house behind to one in front in our small compound, Jean took up a half-hearted stand on the matter but, as a sofa was being turned onto its legs in the new lounge, we found Paul there, appearing from underneath. He just stayed on for four years. Jean took up another firmer stand when Paul went on leave. On his return he took a scruffy room in the Marunouchi Hotel and we went down for dinner and then to his room. Paul looked crestfallen. He was looking for a flat but had not found anything suitable. I did not want to say anything and Jean and I had a desultory conversation in the car on the way home. We did not mention Paul except to say that he looked well. When we got back to the house, Jean looked up the phone book and dialled a number.

"Hello, is that you, Paul? If you want to come back I suppose your room is still empty."

I did not say anything, and just hid behind a magazine. Paul and his gear were back as he joined us for breakfast in the morning.

Paul took his duties seriously. From time to time we would have a crisis with the maids, who had a bad habit of resigning suddenly or indeed not turning up from days off; in these circumstances he would always find out what our plans were and arrange to stay in to look after the girls if we were going out. At another time Jean noticed that the girls were very affluent, buying a mixture of unsavoury looking sweets in profusion from the *tengosan*. *Tengosans* were the itinerant street vendors who went round with an easel, setting up a succession of coloured pictures and telling a story to go with the pictures; they rang their own sounding bells and soon had a group of children standing listening to the story; judging from the pictures their tales contained a good deal of blood and thunder. Large ferocious-looking individuals were frequently lopping off the heads of their foes and other miscreants, there was usually a maiden or two in distress and a prince eventually dealt out justice. I am afraid that with the advent of television, the *tengosans*, members of a worthy and good profession, have become a vanished race.

Jean discovered that Paul was in the habit of ladling out 100 yen notes to Corinna and Alexi, who bought the most revolting sweetmeats from the *tengosans* and the local shops. He was unwilling to give up this pastime and the girls would have been just as upset if

118

he had done so. The problem was solved by me giving Paul their pocket money so that Paul did the actual handing over, though there is little doubt that he continued to augment the amounts. In the East one must learn to save face.

Paul was a chartered accountant and took it upon himself to arrange my tax matters. Owing to the fact that we sent some earnings abroad and divided some US cash, our official yen bank account covered only salaries, rent and the like. Paul was horrified to discover that, by the end of our first year after the Peace Treaty, according to our books Bernard and I owed a mere US$25 in tax for the whole year.

"We will just put some yen in the bank account," said Bernard and I.

"You can't," said Paul. "The bank statements are complete till the end of April."

"What shall we do?" we asked.

"I shall just have to cope with the taxman. I hope it is not Teraokasan, he is a real devil."

A few days later Paul told us he had spent a very unpleasant hour with Teraokasan but that he had finally agreed.

"Sign here," said Paul, shoving a form in front of each of us, "and give me a cheque for nine thousand yen. You are going to have to do much better next year."

"How much do you think it should be next year?" asked Bernard, always one to be on the right side of things.

"Well, you don't want to make it too dramatic. I should think you should aim at about US$300 next year."

"Good," said Bernard, looking relieved.

The Japanese, after the Peace Treaty, modelled their income tax system on American principles. Early on, they had far too few men in the department and they were for the most part hopelessly inexperienced. Like all tax gatherers they learned very fast indeed to become a thorn in the flesh of fellow countrymen and foreigners alike. No quarter is extended nowadays.

A partnership between a Scot, a man who is supposed by reputation to be very careful with money, and a German Jew, by reputation cunning and farsighted in business, should have the potential for enormous gain. The commonly accepted characteristics of these two in combination should produce profit and efficiency. Well, as there was no real competition we could hardly fail to make a profit, but as businessmen we were very inefficient, with a high proportion of bad debts and a good many giveaways. Bernard was far more interested in his medicine than in financial reward and things did not get any better when we recruited a third member, Derek Fair. Derek had been working for United Nations Relief and Rehabilitation in Korea. A New Zealander and a paediatrician, he also was more interested in his medicine than in money. In a practice which was limited in numbers, Derek was always turning up some rare type of case. I well remember him calling me on the intercom to come into his office to see a case of cranio-cleidal dystrophy, which is the only one I have ever seen. It is a congenital condition most noted for the complete absence of the collar bones. It does not do sufferers any harm; in fact they often have the ability to bring the shoulders together in front of the chest so that the shoulders almost touch. This they perform as a parlour trick. This lad, although only four years old, had already discovered this and was only too happy to show it off.

Bernard and Derek were men of utter integrity. To be associated with two such men is rare. Integrity one expects, but they exhibited this quality in its utmost manner. Neither of them would take any action which involved our partnership without considering every aspect of such an action and, above all, they would never do anything to the disadvantage of the others. If there was a chance that I might not agree, the matter would be frankly discussed. Even a mild disapproval was sufficient for them to drop an idea and they would not harp on the subject again.

Once Bernard wanted a more elaborate electrocardiograph apparatus than the one we possessed.

"What is wrong with the one we have?" I asked.

"Nothing is wrong with it, but the one I have in mind is better and more comprehensive," he replied.

I remarked that it would take a long time for such an elaborate machine to pay for itself. Sometime afterwards his wife Susan told me that Bernard had set his heart on the new machine. My mind went back to the brief conversation on the subject and how I had dismissed the idea in a rather cavalier fashion. After all, Bernard's chief interest was cardiology and my knowledge of the intricacies of cardiac diagnosis was rudimentary. I waited for a suitable opportunity.

"Bernard," I said, "you talked to me about a new ECG machine. I know nothing about them and it was a bit high-handed of me to dismiss the idea so quickly. Let's talk about it again."

"No, Gren," said Bernard. "We came to a decision. We are not going back on it."

We both had to curb Derek a bit. Derek was a perfectionist. Although I never saw him take a photograph or indeed show me any pictures he had taken, he was the type of person who, despite the fact that he had the previous month purchased the latest Canon camera, could not resist buying the very latest Nikon. He must either have had one of the world's largest collection of cameras or discarded them by the dozen. I never did find out what he had done with the previous month's model. If you were off for a day or two in the country he was only to happy to lend you a camera, and explain in detail how to use it. He would also like to look at the results of my efforts, which were usually atrocious because I had failed to get some setting correct.

"Mm," he would say on seeing the pictures. There would be a long pause. "Very nice pictures." They were damned by faint praise, which was even more devastating in its impact considering that I had probably only shown him a few of the better ones, withholding the majority which bordered on disastrous. He was well aware of this as any time he lent me a camera he would load it with film, a wise precaution as I would inevitably get the procedure wrong.

With such a person who liked equipment for the equipment's sake, we had to keep a weather eye open; at the drop of a hat he would have purchased for our small laboratory an X-ray machine and equipment designed for use in a large hospital with hundreds of beds. However, a man like him can be relied upon to be up to date with the latest advances in equipment and, provided the apparatus is in fact designed for office use, it may well be much more efficient.

Every now and then he would try to catch us off guard with some suggestion. He would watch our expressions, and if he was greeted with a look of startled horror he would develop his slow smile and change the subject.

Both Bernard and Dick were men of deep culture with well-stocked libraries of both medical and general books. Bernard was not much use as a source of reading material as most of his books were in German. Both my partners were fond of music, owned big record collections and constantly attended concerts. As the Japanese are fanatical in their interests, huge audiences can be guaranteed for any well-known artist or orchestra, so there was a constant succession of top quality performers.

121

There is a tendency amongst people interested in music and art to regard those with different interests as philistines, but my partners never exhibited such an attitude. They realised that John Besford, the dentist, and I were different types of people. Whatever their private thoughts might have been they did not at any time hint of any intellectual superiority. Both Bernard and Derek would on social occasions introduce topics which they knew we were interested in, despite the fact that John needed no encouragement to get started on the subject of his latest enthusiasm, covering the whole matter comprehensively and at considerable length. John could not be faulted. When his interest was aroused in something new he bought books, studied cross references, became an authority, but he would admit straight away that this was new knowledge and a new subject to him. None of it was an irritating pretence of having known these facts for years.

Some months before Derek joined us, the American Chamber of Commerce had decided that the time had come for us to reimburse them for their trouble and financial outlay. The newly-appointed representative of the Chamber came to see me with their statement of accounts. To my horror this amounted to twenty-five thousand US dollars. I took several deep breaths and reminded him of the letter I had sent to E. J. Griffiths voicing my concern about the accounts or lack of them, and furnished them with a record of all the money which had been given to me personally. The representative was taken aback, took my figures and departed. He came back after a few days with the news that the medical sub-committee had convened two lengthy meetings at which my letter was produced. My guess is that they were a little embarrassed that their own fellow national, Tom, seemed to have been the major beneficiary of their bounty. He told me that if I paid them six thousand dollars myself and five thousand from the clinic they would call it square. They did not question my figures. This was a noble and generous act. The balance was not asked for nor was it officially ever mentioned, although the odd remark was made to me off the record from time to time. I wrote them a second letter expressing my gratitude and thanks, to which there was a reply saying they had confidence in us and wished us success in the future; a rider was added that our indebtedness was considered to be totally repaid. This was a typical American act of understanding, fair-mindedness and generosity. It was a gesture which Bernard and I will never forget.

Chapter 17

MONEY

Juggling the currencies — MPCs are recalled and reissued — A very delicate matter — Going round regulations and red tape.

While money plays a part in all our lives, it exercised a disproportionate effect on the lives of foreign residents in Japan. There were really three currencies in circulation; the yen, the American dollar and MPC, short for Military Payment Certificate.

MPC were issued in note form in denominations similar to the American dollar. They were strictly designed and controlled for use on US Army Camps, in the PX or military department stores, the commissaries, the food and provision shops on every base and for paying the occupation civil servants. The largest PX in Japan was situated in what had been the biggest department store in Tokyo, namely Takashimaya, and the PX filled all the building. As many of the commodities of life deemed essential for foreign residents could only be obtained in the PX or commissary, it was mandatory to have MPC despite the fact that this was illegal for civilians. Cigarettes, wines and spirits enjoyed a lively black market and presented no problem, but try going without bacon, cheese, new tyres for your car, a refrigerator, butter that does not taste fishy, Lea and Perrins sauce, or curtain material, to mention only a few of the myriad items of daily living. Possession of MPC, the only currency valid in the military stores, was a necessity. True, the non-military person did not have right of entry but the regulation was so laxly applied that any foreigner just walked in. If you were stopped it was no crime to go in — you were merely turned back. As most of the American forces had only MPC, and never handled yen, they spent the currency freely around town in bars and nightclubs; getting MPC was not too difficult.

Yen was necessary for all one's local purchases. I paid the rent for the house in yen and our staff were paid in yen, but the office rent was paid in dollars and the loan from the American Chamber was in dollars. Such transactions, together with the buying and selling of yen, were concluded in US dollar cheques. As the official rate was Y360 to the dollar and a dollar cheque would get you a rate of Y450, only a saint obeyed the law. At the end of a month one was apt to need yen to settle bills for the house and utilities, with a more constant requirement of MPC for daily living, and dollar cheques forming the reserve. It sounds complicated but really it was not. You soon got to know people who would give a supply of yen for dollars or dollars for yen. On a large scale there were unofficial brokers making a living out of brokerage; but for small amounts, someone in the dining room of the building would accommodate you at the current rate without taking a percentage. As yen were hedged around with all sorts of restrictions, it was customary to realise any profits made in dollar cheques. All this was illegal but was so widespread and indeed, so much of a necessity, that virtually all foreign residents wheeled and dealed in this manner.

We sent out our bills in dollars as many patients did not have a yen bank account. Every now and then someone would pay in yen at 360 to the dollar. This was reckoned to be very sharp practice, if not plain dishonest. Their names were noted and any future service was calculated in dollars but billed in yen at the current market rate. Any complaint about the price going up was met with a scowl or — better tactics — a look of complete surprise. No one would refuse a dollar note but they were not highly desirable. Cheques were the best, and MPC were at a slight discount.

Every now and then without warning MPC would be recalled and reissued in a different colour of note. The military would have to change their notes on that day or explain why not and be confined to barracks. Foreign residents were caught short and the corridors of our building were full of figures scurrying to and fro in efforts to lodge their currency with some privileged source. Ordinary business on that day came to a halt. As the American pharmacy next door to us was allowed to deal in both MPC and yen, I had only to stroll in and lodge my MPC against future purchases.

It was apparently an entertaining sight which unfortunately I never saw, being too busy with my own problems, to see all the bar girls from the bars which surrounded military bases throwing bundles of MPC over the wire around the camp to their GI boyfriends, in the hope that the GI would honour the transaction in one way or another. A profession which usually demands cash before delivery was forced to indulge in the granting of credit on a large scale with no underwriting or collateral. Trust is the basis of all good business.

Another feature of currency was that foreign employees of large concerns had to pay tax on their normal salaries paid in Japan, and the tax rate was very high. As time passed we took in more and more yen, so that I had a surplus. The employees of some of the companies could not live on their nominal yen salary and at the beginning of every month I dropped in for coffee with the wife of one such to give her a fat bundle of notes. In consideration, a set sum of dollars was transferred to my account in San Francisco every month. This system, which did not involve the passage of a cheque, was foolproof. I would receive an agitated phone call if it was difficult for me to make the time for the detour to her home on the first or second day of the month.

There was a charming but diffident lady who came to see me regularly every month. The first time she sat down opposite me she introduced the subject circumspectly and with great caution.

"I hear you might buy yen," she said.

"True, I do sometimes, but usually I am selling."

She appeared crestfallen. She knew other people who would purchase yen but mostly they were in her husband's company, and she was worried that he would get to hear about it. After a little probing on my part she confessed that she saved on the housekeeping as her husband was a spendthrift, and this was the only way she could build up a nestegg for them both. As they were Americans and I was a different nationality, she felt that dealing with me was more secure. Her big innocent eyes looked at me from a lovely face. I succumbed and was happy to oblige. We both came to enjoy our little monthly conspiracy and the secret never leaked out. My reward was to tease her gently with a very slight indiscreet remark when we met at a party. She always got the benefit of any doubt regarding the rate of exchange; a pretty face can launch a thousand ships.

It came almost as a shock to be confronted with a situation where people were apparently forced to abide by the rules. Britain had very strict currency controls and no less than a director of the Bank of England was visiting Japan to conclude a yen-sterling agreement. He brought a secretary, a young girl from England, who almost immediately developed a very bad back and was forced to languish in hospital. Being enfolded in the currency world, it intrigued her to find out what financial advantage accrued to working in a country with similar restrictions and with money which at that time was less desirable than sterling. She looked at me askance when my outline of the methods employed was explained. It was illegal for a resident of Britain to have a US dollar account but not, I pointed out to her, for a semi-permanent resident of Japan, which was how I was classified. I did not have a Bank of England approved Japan sterling account which permitted transfer of sterling to yen, a necessity for trading, although at one time the forms had been sent for my perusal. As the first salvo fired by the questionnaire was to ask for details of your world-wide income, it seemed prudent to consign the form to the wastepaper basket and forget all about it. The longer the Bank of England and any related agencies remained in total ignorance not only of my world-wide income but indeed of my existence, the better.

She must have been steeped in red tape regulations because she returned to the subject frequently. Whether she had confidence in my treatment was not apparent, but what was crystal clear was that she had none in my integrity. Looking back I think I was a little cruel to her; it cannot have been pleasant for her to have been stricken almost immediately on arrival in the exotic East and incarcerated for nearly three weeks in hospital instead of doing her job, and enjoying the sightseeing and different life of the Orient. When she had recovered sufficiently to be discharged to return to the Embassy, where luckily her boss still had a couple more weeks of work, she made one final effort to encourage me to mend the error of my ways.

In exasperation I said to her, "The regulations are damn silly, anybody can poke a hole in them. Why, only the other day I sold five hundred of your precious pounds to an Australian who is now visiting England and he gave me a dollar cheque. He is buying a car, and he benefited by getting the pounds more cheaply, I have benefited with some needed dollars and the British car industry has benefited from another sale."

If my information had been such that through my efforts one of the Royal Navy's destroyers had been sunk, she could hardly have viewed me as a greater saboteur of Merrie England.

She remarked with some satisfaction, "The director told me we are short of yen, so if you do not have a Japan account I don't know if you will be paid for looking after me."

"We will worry about that when the time comes," I replied.

The director himself came to my office to settle the bill.

"I am a bit pushed for yen," he said. "Will a sterling cheque do?"

It was my duty to point out that he was perpetrating a felony by allowing money to be placed in my domestic UK account against a service in a foreign land.

He smiled as he handed me his cheque.

"I know all about that from my secretary. We are out to stop people dealing in thousands; I shall not even embarrass you by asking which bank the cheque will be lodged with. If you don't mind, I would like a receipt to cover my expenses."

We parted the best of friends.

Chapter 18

THE DENTIST AND THE ROCKS

A Japanese house in Aberatsubo — Looking sharp with a shark on screen — The fishermen and the friendly foreigner — A tree transaction — Following up on a patient — In the dental chair — In search of rocks at Odawara — A most expensive footbath.

A woman patient once said to me, "John Besford is the only dentist I know who, on asking you to "rinse please", hands you the cup and makes you think it is champagne!"

John was a man of tremendous enthusiasms. He had been in Britain's team at the Berlin Olympics in 1936 as a backstroke swimmer. He held the 600 metres backstroke world record for nineteen years. He was the first to admit that the record stood for so long because 600 metres is an unusual distance.

For recreation he would go swimming for several hours, covering long distances. One weekend, while engaged in this pursuit, he came across an inlet at Aberatsubo. There was a long narrow arm of the sea, sheltered and inaccessible, where the hillsides descended steeply to the edge of the sea. Scattered around the inlet were several small bays, of which only one had a sandy beach, measuring seventy yards across. The sides of the bay were enclosed by rocky promontories. At high tide the sea came right up to the cliff and at low tide it was a long scramble round the rocks to reach the bay. Behind the beach was a strip of foreshore which itself fronted a small paddy field nestling in the clasp of the cliffs. A steep path descended down the cliff from the fields above. Halfway down was a cave in the cliff front. The mouth of the cave was secured by stout iron doors. Aberatsubo was one and a half hours by car from Tokyo, with the final quarter of a mile a bumpy ride on a track through the fields to a spot at the top of the cliff. The difficulty of access by land and sea made the bay completely private.

John went to the local land office and found he could purchase the strip of foreshore, which was big enough to accommodate a house. The owner of the paddy field would not sell the field, only the foreshore, and declared firmly that the field would always remain a field. There was no question of anyone building a house on the field.

The official in the land office told John that he must be a clever man because just before the war the bay had been marked for the site of a summer house for the Emperor. The war caused the plan to be shelved, and the cove was later used by *kamikaze* pilots — the suicide pilots — in part of their training. The cave had been enlarged and iron doors provided to house their equipment.

John built a small Japanese house there. A wooden verandah, level with the floor of the house, faced the beach. The floors were covered with thick *tatami* mats, which are made of rushes and measure about six feet by three. Two mats alongside make a *tsubo*, a square with sides of about six feet. A *tsubo* is the Japanese measure of land area. All houses are built to a specified number of *tsubo*. Wooden beams for walls and roof are produced in standard lengths which exactly fit across the width of two, four or eight *tsubo*. House construction is fast and cheap, as all the pieces come in certain sizes as though units of a meccano set, being assembled accordingly. Woe betide the ignorant foreigner who insists on a measurement in square feet; he ends up with seventy-three and a half *tsubo*; for the country craftsman, almost insurmountable problems arise and the costs shoot up like a rocket. The front of the rooms looking onto the verandah had *shoji* doors; a *shoji* is a lattice work of wood covered with tough paper. The *shoji* doors slide sideways in a groove on the floor and a slot in the under edge of the overhang of the wall. There are two parallel sets of grooves so that one door can slide behind its neighbour.

You can drop by the carpenter's shop and buy a new *shoji*, take it home, push it upwards into the slot in the wall and let it drop into the floor groove and you have a new wall or door. There is no need to worry about the size. All *shoji* doors in Japan are exactly the same size and their width is the width of a *tatami* mat. If the frontage of your room is eight *tatami* mats wide you need eight single or four double *shoji* doors. It is as simple as that.

Tatami comes in different qualities, but the usual mat is about three inches deep projecting above a wooden frame. When a *tatami* gets a bit worn after ten years or so, it is simply lifted out in its frame and a new one inserted, fitting exactly to the others around it. Everyone must take their shoes off and put on slippers when entering a Japanese house, because shoes damage the *tatami* and bring in dirt. A quick once-round daily with a broom is all that is necessary for a Japanese housewife. *Tatami* is soft and springy underfoot. At night the *futong*, a light mattress rolled up with the bed-clothes, is brought out of a cupboard and spread on the floor. When it is put back in the closet in the morning the room may be bare except for one low table and a pile of cushions in a corner. Housekeeping is economical and delightfully simple. Sitting on a cushion on the floor with your shoes off is something that some foreigners can never get used to, but there is no reason why a foreigner should not put an armchair or two in the room and a carpet over the *tamati*.

After John had got everything suitably established, he looked for new interests. Scuba diving was a natural. It is now a popular world-wide sport but in 1956 it was still in its infancy. Equipment was basic and hard to come by, but by dint of searching, trial and error, he had his own compressor engine, air tanks and guns. He was the first efficient scuba diver in Japan, and his reputation quickly spread. The results were twofold: television appearances and a reputation with the local fishermen. One cold Sunday morning in December a large television team was to arrive from Tokyo with underwater movie cameras and all accessories. John took off in the early morning to plunge in for a reconnaissance; right at the mouth of the bay he encountered a five-foot shark. Any shark under twenty-five feet would have been well advised to get as far away as possible from John Besford; but it lingered and for its temerity got a harpoon in its midriff. The weapon transfixed the shark but did not hit a vital part. It was secured by the harpoon rope, so John towed it back to the boat, fixed the line to the boat and slowly brought the catch back to the beach where the shark remained tethered to the anchored boat, swimming to and fro, apparently unconcerned.

When the television team was ready for action it was easy to obscure the harpoon and line from the camera. Towing the shark into deep water John made a couple of passes to smite the shark with two more harpoons. The whole film lasted fifteen minutes. It was a hit on Japanese TV and excerpts were shown as far away as New York.

The fishermen in the local village soon became aware of the advantages of this friendly foreigner. Like most things in Japan, fishing is highly organised. The fishermen were members of a guild. If you knew them, it was possible to buy privately one or two of their catch, but as a guild their entire catch went three miles to Misaki at the end of the peninsula, to supply bait to the ocean-going fishing schooners that plied in search of tuna amongst the Pacific Islands as far away as the Equator. The Aberatsubo fishermen soon learnt that

THE DENTIST AND THE ROCKS

they could fish in areas of nearby fertile waters that they previously had shunned because their nets had become entangled on the rocky bottom. John's first task at the weekend was to dive to salvage a valuable net or two. Even on a misty day when the cross bearings from the land were invisible the fishermen would direct John's boat to an exact spot, no different as far as we could see from any other patch of water. Down he would go, come back for a line, dive again and in five minutes the net was back on board from an eighty-foot depth. Needless to say, John's standing and prestige with the local village fishermen was immense.

They willingly permitted him to raid their special larder. He was much to sensible to overdo this. A huge net with wide interspaces hung from the surface to the seafloor. It stretched in a straight line a mile seaward to end in a great round bowl of smaller netting some thirty yards across with a three-foot gap where it joined the mile-long big net. The gap was the entrance to a trap. Looking down through goggles you might see a three or four-foot long fish threading its way through the interstices of the big net. When it got to the trap a fish might, of course, turn right and find itself on the outside of the trap but the chances were fifty-fifty that it would incline left and go through the three-foot gap into the trap, there to swim apparently aimlessly round and round. How many found their way out of the gap we do not know but John said he had seen the same fish in the trap for more than twenty-four hours. There might be fifteen or twenty big chaps in the trap, but John was in amongst them like a leopard. He would take only one fish and he always told the headman of the village before he went. The appearance of his boat was recognised from far away but anyone else who ventured there got pretty short shrift from the locals; there were few divers at that time, myself included, efficient enough to do damage. We never discovered why the villagers would leave the trap sometimes for a week and at other times haul it up every day or second day. Generations of experience had dictated the decision; they knew instinctively but could not explain the reasoning.

Many a weekend we spent at Aberatsubo. Jean and my girls would join Mary Besford and their daughter Sherry. The girls went out on John's boat, played on the sand, swam, were in and out of the house in their bare feet, enjoyed alfresco meals and the steaming hot Japanese bath; at night they fell fast asleep in their *futongs*. The girls and their mothers lay strewn across the floor in one room while the men disposed themselves in the other. In the winter John and I would often go down there by ourselves, and get the big square stove, backed by a reflecting sheet of copper, roaring away. We would make determined inroads into the supplies of Old Smuggler. When Ebisu, the British Forces Camp in Tokyo, closed down, John was able to relieve the camp of its entire supply of Old Smuggler Scotch whisky at its duty-free price of about ten shillings or US$1.50 a bottle. The crates were shipped by launch, hauled over the beach by Kimiesan, the village headman, and his helpers and installed in the cave. The iron doors were closed and secured with a padlock. The cave was never burgled, and the supply lasted for four years.

On the sad day when the very last bottle was to be broached, John asked me down.

"It is fitting that you are here, Gren," he said. "After all, apart from myself you have drunk more of it than anybody else!"

We would sit on the floor at the low table, play cards or chess, down the Old Smuggler, occasionally add a log or two to the stove, and listen to the wind howling and the waves crashing against the rocks. When Scrabble was invented we fought contest after contest. John had a huge vocabulary and he would beat me three times out of four. One night I had lost three in a row but near the end of the fourth game I was comfortably in the lead. John laughed a triumphant laugh as he put the letters LITT in front of the word ORAL to make LITTORAL. To my chagrin a double word score put him ahead. With my turn there was little I could do except add S as a plural. He turned the board with a devilish grin, added GAVE to run down below the A of ORAL.

"Out," he said, "One hundred and thirty eight to one hundred and twenty."

"Come on, John," I said, "What the hell is an agave?"

He thrust in the knife. "Didn't they teach you botany at Edinburgh University? It is a plant. As a matter of fact, Gren," he added, giving the knife a determined twist, "the agave is a bush or plant which grows well on the Mediterranean seacoast, or if you prefer the phrase, the Mediterranean littoral."

One day outside our office at Suikosha a truck went by. A huge tree was draped with branches protruding away in front of the cab, with the trunk slanting downwards to beyond the lowered tailgate. A great cone of earth which enclosed the twisted roots hung over the back nearly scraping the ground.

"What is that doing?" John asked me.

"It is coming from a tree farm to be transplanted. There is a tree farm close to my house," I said.

"Really." His interest was immediately aroused and soon he knew far more about tree farms than I. The trees for transplanting are specially doctored; the roots are exposed from time to time and twisted inwards so that the tree, roots and cone of earth can be lifted out and transported to a new site. Most tree farms are family affairs; the tree sold by the farmer may well have been planted by his father many years before. When the tree is replanted, three or four long planks or beams spread outwards from halfway up the trunk to act as supports and are left to help hold the tree in position for about a year, by which time the roots will have taken a firm grip.

It was not long before new trees with their supporting tripods started to appear in the garden of John's home in Tokyo. There were three silver pines in a row, very fine trees already almost thirty feet in height.

John's house in Tokyo had long lateral arms with the short hall and entrance joining the arms, which enclosed a patio facing west. John considered that a tree in the centre of the patio would add grace and provide shade. The tree farm favoured by John was twenty miles out of Tokyo. There was a tree there which he described to me as being exactly right to shade the patio. The bark was a reddish brown, the branches were plentiful, sloping at just the correct angle upwards from the trunk. The size of the tree was perfect. He was determined to buy it. The only snag was that this tree was right outside the farmer's house, had not been cultivated for transplanting, and the farmer liked it. He would not sell it. He did not know John, who gathered his forces for battle.

The preliminary skirmish took place when John and Endosan, his dental mechanic, went out one Saturday to swap yarns with the farmer and drink a little beer and *sake,* the Japanese rice wine. The softening-up process was continued a week later and the all-out grand assault planned for the following Sunday.

John's car was loaded early with bottles of beer, bottles of *sake,* Old Smuggler, Coca Cola for the farmer's daughters, cakes, *obento* boxes of tasty fish morsels, *zushi,* appetizing raw fish, rice, fermented rice, chocolates, a radio, and a record player. Endosan, Haradasan, John's secretary, who was as pretty as a picture, my secretary Onodasan, Fumikosan, the girl dentist, and Sakodasan, our radiographer who was recruited for the day as he had been a law student, all piled in. The day was fine, and everyone sat at a table outside the farmer's house. Beer, *sake* and Old Smuggler went down the hatch, food was consumed in great quantities, the radio was full on, and the record player blared away. John's boisterous laugh and his Japanese expressions with alcoholic fluency echoed back from the trees. Haradasan and Fumikosan allowed the wife and daughter to try on their kimonos amidst giggles and blushes. Endosan got completely plastered and passed out, while Sakodosan was encouraged to stick to beer in the hope that he would remain sober enough to clinch the legal aspects of the proposed sale. Onodasan was the daughter of a Japanese baron and added a somewhat inebriated aura of aristocratic charm — two drinks made her talkative and unsteady on her legs. John was by now the Merry Monarch and the Japanese farmer was about nine points gone on the Beaufort scale. The sale was made and wads of yen changed hands. Sakodosan had lost the letter of formal ratification but no matter, any squiggle of a signature would do. John and his cohorts departed in triumph. In due course I expressed my tremendous admiration of the tree planted in the centre of the patio. No ugly planks supported his arboreal masterpiece but delicate wires ran from a collar round the tree trunk to be secured to the gables of the house.

In the middle of May I saw Jean and my daughters off to Scotland by ship from Yokohama. I watched the white liner go past the end of the breakwater and lingered till she was hull down. They were to be gone for four months. With heavy heart I went to my car and drove home to an empty house. Wanting a distraction I called the Besfords. Mary was home and told me to come round. We sat on the patio to have afternoon tea. I kept shifting my chair to escape the hot afteroon sun and wound up sitting right behind the tree trunk. Getting up I pulled down a branch to look at the leaves. They were numerous but thin and delicate.

I said, "It will be nice when the leaves grow bigger and give some shade."

"Gren," said Mary, "these leaves have been on the tree for two months. John has not said anything, and I dare not mention it but they are no bigger now than they were six weeks ago!"

All mention of trees was taboo. A month later I snooped out into the garden. The patio was empty but round the back, behind a potato patch, stood the prince of trees propped up by four dirty planks.

134

One day John came into my office to tell me that he thought he had a rupture or hernia. His diagnosis was correct and arrangements were made for me to operate. A few days later he came in again and we discussed the operation step by step. He had been reading it up in a textbook of operative surgery, and apparently my description was satisfactory.

At one point he said, "I am glad you mentioned that. The books says it is most important."

I said, "John, if you are all that interested we can give a spinal anaesthetic and you can watch it all in the reflection in the overhead operation light." This was agreed upon.

The great day came. John had been given a fairly large pre-operative sedation, the spinal anaesthetic was administered, the operative field painted with antiseptic, and towels arranged round the incision area and over the screen in front of his face. I ascertained that he could see the operative field reflected in the overhead lamp.

Early on, a small skin artery spurted for a second or two before it was clamped off, providing a moment of drama. I kept up a running commentary for his benefit. The sac of the hernia was identified, cleared from surrounding coverings, and isolated up to the neck of the sac. The sac was then twisted several times upon itself to constrict the neck. At this point a suture is inserted through the neck to tie off the sac, and the redundant sac cut off beyond the suture.

"Well, John," I said, "I am just about to suture the sac at the neck here. Then we start the repair." There was no answer. I looked over the top of the screen. The premedicative sedation had worked too well and he was fast asleep.

On the first post-operative day he was sitting on a chair looking out of the window.

"Look here, Gren," John asked, "what is being done for me here that could not be done at home? You can see me by coming upstairs from the office twice a day without trouble." He was living at that time in an apartment above our office.

I outlined the reasons why he should stay in hospital, although I knew I was on a losing wicket; he went back to the flat at Suikosha. Next morning John was again looking out of the window of the flat at a glorious sunny day.

"See you this evening, John," I said on leaving. I was in error. In the evening only the maid was in the flat. Dr Besford had gone to his beach house.

At home I said to Jean, "Do you mind, dear, if we cancel our arrangements for tomorrow? I am paying a surprise visit to Aberatsubo after lunch to give Dr J. C. P. Besford absolute hell."

I left the office early at noon and, without waiting for lunch, drove down past the Yokusha Navy Base and across the fields to park my car at the top of the cliff. A glance showed me that there was no boat hauled up on the beach; possibly the boat boy had taken it round for repair. The house was wide open but no one was home.

Going into the kitchen to make myself a sandwich, the first thing that arrested my attention was a bundle of gauze, sticking plaster and a pair of scissors laid neatly on the sideboard. Could it be that the dressing on his wound might get wet and a new dressing might be needed? The second thing I noticed was that in addition to the bottles of Asahi beer there were two bottles of Kirin beer, my favourite. A surgeon should follow up his patients. Had John had an inkling that his surgeon might follow him down? He would not expect me to leave Tokyo till after the office closed at one o'clock and lunch would last till half past one, so three in the afternoon would be the earliest he would expect me. If so, his planning had miscarried. A quick scramble to the edge of the headland showed an empty bay. There was time to sunbathe on the veranda with the beer and sandwiches, but my ears were cocked for the sound of a boat's engine.

Just after half past two the chug chug of a marine diesel sounded from round the corner giving me ample time to go into the house and adjust two *shoji* doors to leave a gap of an inch or two, through which I could see the beach unobserved.

The boat came into the cove and grounded on the sand, only a few yards away as it was high tide. John had swimming trunks on, and the boat boy held the tiller. John got out to stand in the water, reached into the boat for his flippers and harpoon gun, bent and lifted out two *ishidai*.

The *ishidai* is a black fish with grey stripes. It is flat on the sides and thin if seen from above or head on. The two John held were about standard size, some twenty inches long. It is an inquisitive and fearless fish often coming right up to a skin diver to look at him. You can almost nudge the point of the harpoon against its generous flank, and it is very easy to shoot. However, there is one feature about shooting *ishidai* — they are always at least forty feet below the surface.

At this point I walked onto the beach. John had the decency, like a schoolboy caught stealing apples, to start to put the *ishidai* behind his back. He did not complete the movement, knowing that he was caught red-handed. For once he was bereft of speech.

"Pull your trunks down and let me look at the wound," I commanded. He did so. There was no dressing, just the ladder of seven or eight black silk skin sutures.

"Gren," he said, "you put saline on wounds. Sea water is sterile."

"We put normal saline on wounds. Seawater is hypertonic saline. Did it not hurt?"

"Not at all. Well, it did a bit when I was climbing back into the boat. I had to get the boat boy to give me a hand."

I said sternly, "John, don't blame me if anything goes wrong. There must be damn few surgeons who have a patient who has been at least forty feet down — and don't deny it — on the third post-operative day. Still, the wound looks healthy enough."

The sheepish look had left him and he grinned at me. He was his old self. "Come along in and have a drink. I am sure nothing will go wrong."

Nothing did go wrong. He is still in great shape some twenty years later.

Impressed by the success of my surgery, John determined to do me a favour in return. His interest and enthusiasm finally came to rest on my wisdom teeth. Despite the fact that my wisdoms had grown through the gums some fifteen years previously without doing me any noticeable injustice, despite no visible signs of my jaw becoming malformed, despite my other teeth seeming to live in perfect harmony with them, John developed an acute loathing for these harmless chewers and painted a horrible picture of what would happen if I insisted on retaining them. No one could hold out forever against such a malevolent menace to my appearance, health and general welfare.

The left lower came out without trouble; I do not remember having any pain or discomfort. On the other hand, I do not remember gaining any benefit either. I managed to hold onto the right lower for a further month or two.

In those days that nasty four-letter word which is now bandied about three times on every page of modern literature was a word I reserved for moments of extreme provocation. I might utter it if I got a flat tyre at midnight, could not find the jack and discovered that my torchlight battery was dead. One uses it so frequently nowadays for trivial mishaps that there remains no satisfactory expletive for a serious situation.

I never heard John swear. When things were bad he said "Brother," and when the crisis was of monumental proportions he raised the tension to fever pitch with "Oh, Brother!"

He got me in the chair for the second time. The local anaesthetic was working very well and I felt nothing except the ache one gets from keeping one's mouth wide open for an interminable time. He seemed to experience more difficulty than with the left lower molar three. Like all dentists the number of objects they can insert into your mouth and expect you to retain there passes ordinary belief — a sucker apparatus, pads, retaining clamps, clamps which hold your jaw open, prongs, probes and chisels which they euphemistically call osteotomes, plus two or three of their fingers.

John had been working away for some twenty minutes before he said "Brother."

Some cause for alarm! Mine.

A few "Brothers" later and he seized a scalpel, of a size which personally I would have reserved for a limb amputation done under adverse circumstances demanding tremendous speed. The scalpel found its way through the impossible array of foreign matter in my mouth and after some thirty seconds John said "Oh Brother!"

I just closed my eyes and gripped the arm rests.

An eternity passed.

"Well, there we are, Gren," he said. I opened my eyes and he waved the tooth in front of me.

"Looks clean as a whistle, but Brother, it wasn't easy."

For a week or two odd bits of bony tissue which I presumed to be parts of my mandible were extruded from time to time. When I come to think of it, I did not feel any particular benefit from parting with my right lower molar three either.

The farmer who owned the paddy field behind the house at odd times planted a crop of vegetables there. The abundant growth contrasted with the few plants clinging to a precarious existence on the foreshore. The difference presented by the meagre garden at John's seaside house was a challenge which could not be met until Professor Azabuki hove on the scene. The Professor headed a university department of agriculture. He was an authority on

Japanese gardens, soil properties and plants. Only certain species of flowers and plants could grow in the mixture of sand and earth located so close to the sea. He mapped out a course of action to establish a beautiful garden. Because of the rarity of the plants, windbreak hedges, fertilisation needs and expert care, the cost would be astronomical, far greater than that of the land and house combined. John thought about it, and reluctantly came to the conclusion that the expense was not justified.

He was downhearted and met with Azabukisan to tender his apologies. Azabukisan was also downcast and pondered the problem with wrinkled brow. An air of gloom prevailed. Suddenly Azabukisan's countenance cleared.

"Why don't you put some rocks round the house?" he asked.

"But there are rocks everywhere," said John.

"Ah so. Not the right kind of rocks. The rocks used in a Japanese garden are special rocks. The best place for them near here is Odawara."

John told me about this with a hearty laugh and the subject was dismissed, or so I thought. A small seed had been planted at the back of his mind and the only extraordinary thing about it was that it lay dormant for so long in such a fertile matrix. It must have been at least two months before Mary casually remarked to me that her husband had gone off for the day to Odawara. I did not have to wait long before the subject of rocks was mentioned in the office.

Lake Hakone empties through a series of gorges tumbling down three thousand feet to form a river entering the sea at Odawara, which is forty miles south of Tokyo.

The rocks in the estuary and final mile of the river are round and of different sizes. Their value, which can be high, depends on their size, degree of roundness and colour; some are grey, others have a brown or greenish hue. A rock fancier cannot just go and take a few. Azabuki, though an authority on their aesthetic properties, was no geologist but his guess that they took a few hundred years to form was probably correct and the supply was not inexhaustible. Their purchase was controlled by a franchise and they did not come cheap. John, of course, was under starter's orders for a new project.

"How about a trip to Odawara?" he asked me.

At first my inclination was to accept, but a moment's reflection told me that my interest in rocks would wane after half a hour, by which time John and Azabuki would just be getting into their stride.

True, I could go to a bar I knew of where there were two cute Japanese barmaids. It is one thing to break the journey to Hakone for ten minutes over a couple of beers and swap pleasantries in halting Japanese and sign language, but it is another to cope with several hours of their company. I declined the invitation.

Between them they selected nine small rocks about the size of a football, two medium ones two feet in diameter, and the pièce de resistance, a rock the height of a man and weighing over a ton. The big fellow was almost a perfect sphere except for a depression twenty inches across and three or four inches deep. It would sit firmly on the depression, thought John. The cost of the large rock accounted for most of the total price which was about US$250.

"How are you going to get them over the fields and down the cliff?" I asked.

"We are not. We are hiring a lighter and a tug. It is all arranged for Saturday, when luckily it is high tide in the afternoon. It is only twenty miles across Sugami Bay and the tug will get the lighter there and onto the beach when the tide is in. The headman in the village will get some chaps to help with the unloading."

"Bit expensive, all that," I said.

"Well, not really. The tug is not one of those which pulls liners in and out, it is more of a glorified motor boat with the captain and one boy as crew. The lighter hardly warrants such a title. Kimiesan and his lads will offload for nothing."

On Monday morning, John said, "There has been a sort of hitch. We got all the small ones off and even the two medium size were not difficult, but the big one presented a problem. I don't think that Kimiesan was quite prepared to tackle such a monster rock. However, they got some poles and ropes and fashioned a few slings. There was a lot of talk and discussion."

I could imagine the indrawing of breath with which the Japanese contemplate an unusual problem. *"Ah so desuka"*, *"Ayah"* and other equivalents of the English "Gosh", "Heave-ho", "To you and from me" etc., would have been bandied about. Grunts and groans would accompany the efforts.

"Anyway," said John, "they got it raised about two feet when something happened. One of the ropes slipped and the rock crashed back onto the bottom of the lighter. The trouble was that it went right through the bottom, water poured in and the whole thing sank. It is not a total loss of course, as it was already aground at the bow but the stern went down."

"Did the captain go down with his ship?" I enquired.

John was not very happy with my levity.

I had hit on a sore point. The captain had offered no advice or help, but had remained aloof from the whole operation, only coming into action after disaster had struck. Firstly, the captain would take his tug back to Odawara; secondly, he would hope to return to pick up the tow; thirdly, although Kimiesan and the locals would perform jury repairs for the trip back, the lighter would have to be docked at Zushi for professional attention and lastly, there was the Japanese equivalent of demurrage. One cannot better the Oxford dictionary's description of the term demurrage: "Rate or amount payable to ship-owner by charter for failure to load or discharge ship within the time allowed." The whole cost of the venture was rising by leaps and bounds. Negotiations with the captain were, I gather, quite protracted. Kimiesan and the villagers would effect repairs between high tides and would not charge for this service, but the captain was more venal.

John thought of sending a minion on the lighter for the return trip as he considered that the captain might well blame Kimiesan for poor repairs, sabotage the lighter somewhere in Sugami Bay and claim for total loss. John was dissuaded. The lighter reached Zushi without further mishap.

Now the rocks were assembled above the tide line in a neat pyramid, awaiting the expert attention of Professor Azabuki who would be down during the next week to arrange for their permanent placing in true artistic fashion, in accordance with the highest levels of Japanese aesthetic garden culture. Kimiesan & Co. would be needed again for the actual labour as Professor Azabuki was the brain power, but the job of handling, shoving and heaving was beneath his dignity. The Professor indicated that it might take a day or two and we presumed that from time to time he would stand back like an artist surveying his canvas, possibly rearranging the order, and trying alternate settings until perfection was achieved.

It was not in John's nature to dwell on misfortune. True, the operation had now become very expensive but, putting these thoughts from his mind, he was afire by Friday to rush down to inspect Professor Azabuki's handiwork. On reaching the top of the cliff he halted. When Balboa, the Conquistador, climbed a peak in Panama and discovered the ocean beyond, in the words of the poet, he "gazed at the Pacific with a wild surmise". John's stocky, robust figure would have done credit to a conquistador; he too gazed down with a wild surmise but it was for a different reason — there was nothing to see at all. His first thought that the rocks had been purloined was dismissed in view of the difficulties of the transport problem. As he hurried down the path and alongside the house, he saw some of the small rocks projecting from the soil in an orderly line; rounding the corner to the front he spied a rock rising to knee height a step from the verandah. Like an iceberg, nine-tenths was out of sight. The great rock was mostly buried and on its upper surface was the small depression. Professor Azabuki thought it would make an admirable foot bath and so it came to pass, in the course of time, that guests would stand for a hallowed moment in the few inches of water, there to wash the sand off their feet before stepping onto the verandah. By far the most artistic of all foot baths had been fashioned and John had qualified again for the Guinness Book of Records. He had just created the world's most expensive footbath!

Chapter 19

THE PILOT

Turks throw coal at bridegroom — Maintaining the supply of booze — What's a fee between friends? — A suitcaseful of money — A trip to the Bank of England.

I first met Dave Lampard when he came to my office in Shanghai. At that time he was a pilot with Hong Kong Airways, a subsidiary of BOAC. Their routes were limited to those between Hong Kong, Shanghai and Canton. Dave was considering resigning to join CAT, an airline which has been mentioned earlier. The names of the airlines operating in China could lead to confusion, CAT, CNAC, CATC, standing respectively for Civil Air Transport, run by General Chennault, China National Aviation Corporation, the national carrier, and China Air Transport Corporation, a quasi-official line.

Dave took the plunge and became, as far as I know, the only British pilot to join CAT. Whether ultimately he would have been better off to have worked his way up the ladder to senior captain with BOAC is questionable; there is little doubt that he would have succeeded as I never heard any pilot in his or any other airline have anything but praise for his flying ability. Set against this, his life would have been less interesting.

When the Nationalists were driven from the mainland, they held for a time the semi-tropical island of Hainan, situated a few miles offshore, not far from North Vietnam. Hainan is a large island, only a few square miles less in extent than Formosa, or Taiwan as it is now called.

CAT was an airline that prospered in times of trouble. It flew every mission, except combat, connected with a country at war. When China came under Communist control and Hainan was also threatened, the reason for CAT's existence had gone. The General gathered his pilots and told them what they already knew: business for CAT was at a standstill and pay would end abruptly. The pilots were given round-the-world air tickets and advised to get their American Airline Transport Rating, known as ATR. Dave, with a group of his friends, went to Milwaukee to attend ground school for the ATR examination and would have gone on to the flying school but for the fact that one evening Dave was caught in the Chief Instructor's office with the Chief's secretary under rather compromising circumstances. The whole group considered that a strategic retreat to St. Louis was prudent. CAT members were well used to rapid decisions regarding retreats and withdrawals. Their stay in St. Louis was not marred by any such untoward incidents and they all got their ATR.

Dave went back to his family in England. He enjoyed himself there but boredom was threatening to set in when Bill Welk passed through London. They both had the unexpended part of their round-the-world tickets and it took little to persuade Dave to head back for the Far East. As Bill and Dave were sipping beer in Beirut the news came through of the invasion of South Korea. Among CAT members, the decision to advance could be made as quickly as to retreat and they got the first booking to Hong Kong.

CAT were back in business, contracting with the US Air Force for thirty planes to ferry supplies to Korea. There were not anything like thirty planes available but the General started negotiations for some of the seventy DC3s and C46s parked at Kaitak in Hong Kong. There was a legal wrangle between Chiang Kai-shek, the Communists, CNAC and CATC as to ownership. The wrangle was not resolved for many months and CAT only managed to scrape together a few planes, far short of the thirty required, so the US Air Force was getting short change for its dollar. A little difficulty like this was no problem to CAT; they hired some painters and nightly new numbers appeared on the tails, convincing the military of the size of the fleet. This ingenious but simple stratagem was so successful that in the future not only numbers but companies, national flags and emblems came and went with bewildering speed and frequency to suit whatever emergency happened to be on hand; the main difficulty was the production of accurate stencils.

Dave was shot straight off as airline station manager at Iwakuni, an Australian base in Japan. Being British and ex-Royal Air Force, he was very acceptable to the Australians, and Dave was good at human relations. He never criticised a nationality but was a master at taking the mickey out of them in such a way that they were not sure if they were being fooled, criticised or praised. His finger would land unerringly on a sensitive spot and it was nearly all the truth.

While at Iwakuni he met his future wife, Naila Gizatullen, who was Turkish. Long before the Russian revolution had caused the tide of White Russians to flood into China, a small group of Turks fleeing from persecution wandered across Siberia to end their exodus in Japan. These people were akin to the people of Southern Russia. The women had the white skin and golden hair of the Georgians; in fact, they probably were Georgian, but a sect worshipping Islam rather than Russian Orthodoxy. This was the reason for their long trek to form a small close-knit community of one or two hundred in Kobe. They maintained their identity, religion, and patois Turkish speech. They did not approve of their daughters marrying infidels, be they Christian, Buddhist or Shinto.

Naila and David eloped. She was eighteen. They had a Mohammedan as well as a Christian ceremony. Naila sat on the floor of the car while travelling between holy places in case some vigilant Turk spotted them. When all was signed and sealed they returned to break the news to the Gizatullen family. Uproar broke out. Turkish reinforcements from nearby houses arrived and Allah's name was invoked with increasing frequency and volume. The Turkish forces, worked up to a mass hysteria, commenced battle, pelting David with lumps of coal.

"Go out to the front, Naila. Courtnay is waiting in the car," said Dave. "I will draw their fire."

Dave retreated through the house and out through the back with chunks of coal whizzing by his head and crashing against the walls. He suffered a few direct hits with smaller pieces.

"And do you know, Gren," he told me, "it wasn't coal but anthracite." For some reason that he has never explained, the bombardment was more heinous because it was not good plain coal but anthracite. Turkish tempers soon cooled and in a year or two Dave had inherited a good bit of responsibility not only for Naila, but for the whole Gizatullen family, who number some five younger ones as well as Ma and Pa.

The newlyweds moved to Tokyo and Dave went back to flying. In the initial confusion and surprise of North Korea's attack, some areas of supply were overlooked. One of these was the maintenance of a sufficient supply of booze for various Officer and NCO clubs. Several enterprises made efforts to fill this gap, one firm in particular being very successful. The two American owners did well and their expert knowledge allowed them to repeat the process in Vietnam, making them very rich men.

As Dave, being British, was occasionally classifed as a security risk, the innocent job of flying three times a week from Tokyo to pick up a cargo in Iwakuni and on to several airfields in Korea became his "milk run". Initially all went well with cases of liquor assigned to specific clubs, but as news of the mercy flights spread, posses of military men met the plane to buy a crate or two right off the plane. As formidable generals and more fearsome top sergeants had ordered their men not to return to their units without the goods, they were not averse to enforcing requests with drawn pistols. Dave was given the task of ensuring that the goods were given to the correct consignees against invoices. This responsibility, added to the hazards of transporting the stuff, resulted in his receiving a small commission as a reward from the grateful owners for each successful mission. On Mondays, Wednesdays and Fridays, Dave took off for his return trip. Everyone profited, both the givers and the receivers.

The operation had almost biblical overtones, and Dave was back home in time for his pre-dinner cocktail. But a CAT pilot did not always have such a simple, rigid timetable; urgent flights and missions would turn up now and then, but none of the pilots were sticklers for the rules of hours of flying or cramping restrictions. They were a loosely joined brotherhood with a marked *esprit de corps*. If the plane had the fuel range, it did not matter where the mission was or what it was; the pilots would go at a moment's notice.

Somewhere at this time these pleasant duties were interrupted. Dave was assigned to fly a CAT DC4 leased to the newly formed Korean National Airways; the change of flags and company was legal this time. Korean National was run by a Captain Shinn, a Korean who had flown with the Japanese Navy. After several tiffs with Dave over operating and other matters. Captain Shinn asked CAT to replace him. They obliged with a 250-lb. pilot known as Earthquake McGoon. One week later Shinn asked for Dave back. No one shed any tears when the body of Shinn was found face down in a small tributary of the Han River. Korean National ceased its existence, waited a while to be reborn, and Dave returned to the milk run. I was happy to know he would be home on certain mornings at his house, a convenient stop near the hospital.

One morning I answered the telephone.

"Hello Gren, Dave here. Look, I don't expect you to tell me how to fly an aeroplane, but I have been reading it up in *Pears Encyclopaedia*. I reckon I have appendicitis, and acute appendicitis at that."

"Rubbish, Dave, but I am coming round straight away to dispel your fears," I replied.

Having examined him, I said, "I must apologise for casting doubt on your clinical acumen. Your diagnosis is 100 per cent correct. I shall try to get you a south facing room in the hospital so you can see your house and garden from the window."

A day or two after the event, Dave asked, "I suppose you are going to charge me a big, fat fee?"

"I have not made up my mind, but if I do render an account it will probably be a token one unless you are rude to me. Rudeness puts the fee up."

"I should jolly well think it should be a token. Under the guise of conveying bulletins regarding my health to Naila you pay prolonged visits to my house twice a day and the amount of refreshment you consume must be equal to any honourable surgeon's fee. I have been watching you through binoculars."

"As you can leave hospital tomorrow I will bring Jean along this evening so that she and Naila can sit out in the garden and you can watch the household bills going up."

In the evening I took along a bottle of Dimple Haig. As we sat on the lawn I held the bottle high in the air. The phone rang. "It is Dave for you, Gren," said Naila.

"Hello, struck by a long-delayed conscience you have brought your own supply, I see."

"Don't you believe it, Dave. The bottle was empty and I poured some of yours into it. It is a Dimple Haig bottle because, even at this range, the shape is easy to identify. Of course, your stuff is not as good as Dimple but it is adequate. Good-bye, see you tomorrow morning."

When their second child was born I had been pressed into service to conduct the delivery. It was touching how my friends reposed their confidence in a surgeon's very occasion skill as an *accoucheur*. I always remembered the words of my old professor when I was a student.

"The mark of a good obstetrician is one who can exhibit boundless patience and masterful inactivity."

The evening of the day of delivery was celebrated by Dave, Duncan Fraser and myself at the Latin Quarter, Tokyo's plushest night club.

"I suppose I had better pay you for your work, Gren," said

Dave, "although you only made it in time by the skin of your teeth. How much do you want? I have my dollar cheque book here."

"Oh," I said. "Give me a hundred bucks."

As by that time we had been in the Latin Quarter for quite some time, the bill for the evening appeared. Dave gave it to Duncan, Duncan pushed it across to me, and in a moment of weakness, I paid.

"Being obstetrician to the Lampard family has left me in debt by about fifteen dollars," I said.

Years later, both Duncan and Dave still refer to this with evident glee and pleasure.

The saga ended when Guy was born.

"You were round at the hospital by the time I put the phone down, Gren. Frightened of losing your fee, I suppose?"

"You are dead right," I said. "Furthermore, any celebrations are being conducted in your house."

It was Dave who involved me in the affairs of another CAT pilot, Eric Dollar. Eric had married a Chinese film star named May Lin, a girl of many talents. Together, May and Eric started a nightclub in Tokyo named the Marco Polo. One of its better attractions was the organ, played by Eric's father. The nightclub was one of the first to start up in Tokyo after the war. A shadowlike figure, Tommy Shin, held a vague managerial position in the background of the club. After a period of initial success, several things started to go wrong and Eric was forced to go to the club in the late evening to make sure of getting his fair share of the takings. Unfortunately, Eric's flying duties often meant that he was away from Japan for several days, and no satisfactory explanation of financial settlements made during his absences could be elicited. The marital affairs of May and Eric started to deteriorate because the relations of May and Tommy Shin — a fellow Chinese — raised many doubts in Eric's mind. Things went from bad to worse both with the Marco Polo and the marriage, until Eric found himself involved as the plaintiff in a divorce action on the grounds of infidelity. This was hard on Eric, as May Lin was famous for the liberality with which she distributed her favours.

Eric and his Japanese attorney attended the divorce court and Eric listened to torrents of Japanese of which he understood not one word. After a long hearing the court reached a decision, and Eric and his attorney walked out.

"Congratulations," said Eric's attorney. "You are now a free man."

Eric had already assimilated this information but he asked his attorney if there had been any financial settlement.

The attorney coughed a couple of times and said, "Yes."

"How much?" enquired Eric.

The attorney coughed again. "Forty-five million yen."

A rapid calculation revealed this to be some one hundred and eight thousand US dollars.

"Well," said Eric, "I don't have eight thousand, much less the other hundred thousand."

May Lin then appropriated Eric's new motor car in part payment, but by organising a masterly raid Eric recovered his car and secretly garaged it at a friend's house. Eric also visited the Marco Polo to remove the reeds from the organ, thus rendering it ineffective, striking a rearguard blow against one of the club's attractions.

May Lin disappeared from the Tokyo scene, returning to Hong Kong. Eric went to their apartment to find if there was anything he could salvage from the wreckage. In a corner cupboard he found a locked suitcase which, when opened, was found to contain two thousand pounds sterling in ten and twenty pound notes. Such notes had been withdrawn from circulation early in World War II. It was natural for Eric to turn to Dave, as an Englishman, for advice and help in the problem of realising this tangible asset. The first move was for Dave to post one note to his bank in London, who replied with a terse communication that the sending of bank notes through the mail was illegal.

However, a questionnaire requiring completion was included, with the advice to write and send it to the Bank of England. Eric and Dave produced a letter explaining how May had sold an apartment in Shanghai and received the notes in part-payment. This was accurate as it happened, but impossible to prove as Shanghai was now under Communist rule. The letter went on to say that Eric believed the British were honourable, and had heard that the Bank of England was the safest and most reliable financial institution in the world; he merely wanted to redeem some of the bank notes they had issued. The Bank wrote back saying they had swallowed the story, but forebearing to mention that it caused indigestion. There were instructions on delivering them by sealed package through the auspices of the British Embassy. As I was going to the United Kingdom it seemed simpler to arm me with the correspondence and the notes.

Should one deem it necessary to visit the Bank of England one is well advised to dress appropriately. A dark suit, a Homburg hat and a rolled umbrella is the standard uniform, as I realised the moment I crossed the threshold. Although my sports jacket and slacks were of sombre hues and conservatively cut, they immediately earned the obvious disapproval of the doorman, and a faint hint of this disapproval hung in the air throughout my visit. The Bank of England is not like any other bank; there is no counter across which you present a cheque. One's business is dealt with on a theoretical plane, and unless the business concerns sums of several millions, one is apt to get short shrift.

The man into whose presence I was eventually ushered did nothing to dispel the aura of disfavour. In fact, his whole attitude suggested that I had intruded and introduced a nasty smell into the hallowed precincts, and the sooner I was gone the better and good riddance at that. He was too well-mannered to express any doubt as to my credentials or the veracity of my statements and I pointed out that my function was that of a messenger. For a moment I considered saying that I was like Mercury, the messenger of the Gods, but heavy-handed attempts at humour would have been out of place. It was a relief to emerge into the diesel fumes of London and prepare to beat a hasty retreat to the cleaner air of Scotland.

The promised letter arrived from the Bank. It was terse and final. "We have examined the Bank of England notes of the following denominations and serial numbers. All the notes have been found to be forgeries and have been destroyed." I wrote to Dave of the failure of my mission.

"The trouble was," said Dave, "Eric never believed me."

Chapter 20

LIFE IN JAPAN

*Coping with rent increases — The Ryans next door — Water problems
— A lawn is covered with logs and oil drums.*

Living in Japan was essentially a matter of compromise, and no
feature demanded this concession more than housing. Large
international companies could afford to buy land to build houses for
their staff. Lesser mortals were forced to rent. The housing
advertisements would quote the phrase "semiwestern style". Such a
description covered a multitude of deficiencies.

Our landlord, Mr Tamura, had two houses in a small compound.
He had enlarged the lounge of one of these and installed a fireplace
of his own design which did not work. The smoke did not come out
of the top of the chimney, but entered the room instead. After
repeated modifications we installed a whole fireplace unit and
chimney ordered from an American mail order firm. Whether the
chimney was at fault or whether the electrical wiring was to blame we
did not discover, but eventually the house was partially burned down
one autumn day when the fire was lit. The fact that the house did not
go up like a torch was no doubt due to the unseasoned wood used as
a supporting lattice work frame for the new walls of the lounge. The
layer of material on the outside of the house, together with the
plaster of the walls, resulted in a thickness of about one inch, and the
pattern of the wood lattice work stood out clearly on the inside walls.
Before the second winter we applied a layer of grass paper. This did
not entirely obscure this pattern, but did serve to provide some
insulating properties in a design which seemed to have been inspired
to conduct heat from the room.

Tamurasan had been in Britain on an undisclosed mission before
the war. He prided himself on two things: his fluent English and his
man of the world business acumen. To satisfy this "businessman"
urge he would attend my office and that of my next door neighbour
to collect the rent rather than come to our houses. He considered our
offices to be in the hub of the Tokyo business world and he always
carried a brief-case which probably contained his lunch. The image of
the suave businessman was dented by the fact that he only had two

suits, both of which were of thick tweed and looked as though they had been bought at a farmer's jumble sale some ten years previously; the suits had the appearance of never having been pressed by their present owner. The image was further marred because he never had all the flybuttons done up; there was the faint excitement of a lottery draw in estimating how many would be unbuttoned when he was ushered in. The average was between two and three and it was a red-letter day when only one was showing. He always indulged in some man-to-man chatter, occasionally introducing a risqué story. As this was conducted in his "fluent" English it would have been entertaining had one been able to decipher more than one word in five.

For some time my next-door neighbour, Frank Ready Junior, and I had been expecting Mr Tamura to introduce the subject of raising our rents, which we knew had fallen behind the general standards; we had agreed to accept a modest increase. Tamurasan delayed his approach much longer than we anticipated, and when he did broach the subject it coincided exactly with the seven per cent Frank and I had thought acceptable. So when I concurred with only a token resistance to the demand he was taken aback, but in a spirit of good fellowship paused at my office door on his way out.

"I knew you were a cricketman," he said.

"I beg your pardon, Tamurasan," I replied.

"All Englishmen are good cricketmen," he replied, and departed.

It dawned on me that he was referring to the English expression, "It is not quite cricket," indicating sharp practice or faintly dishonourable behaviour.

Poor Tamurasan had a great shock when he proceeded forthwith to interview Frank Ready. When he found that, although Frank was American, he was also a good cricketman, he had a heart attack in the outer office. He never recovered completely from the heart ailment and succumbed soon afterwards, leaving Frank and me to deal with a new Tamurasan, his daughter. The daughter had no pretensions to being a tycoon but had greater business acumen, introducing the subject of a further rent increase at her first visit. As Tamurasan the second was far from attractive in appearance and disposition, it helped Frank and me to harden our collective hearts and fight a spirited rearguard action.

Apart from his fireplace inspiration, Mr Tamura was very proud of the basin and toilet he installed off the upstairs master bedroom. The only snag was that the water pressure was insufficient to produce even a drop of water. When this was pointed out he suggested that water be brought up in buckets. This seemed a poor arrangement and once more it was up to the tenant to rectify matters. With my lack of knowledge of hydraulic engineering, I thought the problem could be met by having a pump to fill a tank placed under the roof, but such was not the case; it would have been far too simple. The water engineer consulted to deal with the matter poured scorn on the idea, and in time a concrete tank was sunk outside the back door as a reservoir. A small shed was constructed to house an electric pump of formidable proportions which, by means of an elaborate demand valve, sprang into action with an alarming mighty roar whenever the basin upstairs was filled or the toilet flushed. The gas company installed a water heater in another small shed fixed to the wall. As the wind whistled through the shed the pilot light would blow out, so it was fortunate that it was outside and the gas could escape into the open air. Several months elapsed before these two pieces of mechanism were declared operational, after vast expense had been incurred. Everyone attended the first trial of the upstairs toilet. Gingerly the handle was depressed. An interval elapsed followed by gurgling and hissing sounds. Then suddenly a huge volume of boiling water gushed into the pan, filling the room with steam; hygienic no doubt, but wasteful of gas, so further modifications to the plumbing system were undertaken.

Our first next-door neighbours were Bill and Kate Ryan. Although everyone else called him Bill, his wife was never heard to use his first name. She always referred to him and addressed him simply as Ryan. Bill was from Chicago and Kate from Boston. They arrived with five children, and two years later moved to another house with eight, most of whom had red hair. At one time or another they were all treated by me, and it was an unwritten rule that consultations in the house were free, but serious matters needing an office visit were paid for. However, the decision to seek medical advice was not always subject to parental approval. On one occasion four small girls burst into the bathroom to show me a cut finger which I was able to clean up for closer inspection by immersing the hand in the bathwater in which I was already sitting.

When Kate became pregnant for the seventh time it was decided that she knew far more about conducting both the pregnancy and

153

labour than I, but nevertheless, at least nominally, I was appointed obstetrician. Sometimes over a Scotch and soda I would suggest that while I considered it an honour and testimonial that she should come to me, possibly an official visit to my office for some sort of a check-up might be advisable. My duties as an obstetrician were being sadly neglected, and negligence can be construed as malpractice. Kate was far too busy. In the fullness of time Ryan woke me one morning to announce that things were on the way. We proceeded to the hospital in convoy and were just in time to get Kate into the labour room to deliver a fine boy. The anaesthetic, which had hardly been properly started, was stopped and Kate woke up to be congratulated on a son. This pleased her, as apart from the eldest, Timmy, there had been a succession of girls. While we were enjoying a feeling of mutual accomplishment I put my hand with the skilled obstetrician's touch on the abdomen. It seemed to be about the same size as before.

"Kate," I said, "I think there is another in there."

"Oh no!" she said, "that is impossible."

"Well, if it is not another it must be a bust of Julius Caesar." I do not think Kate appreciated this sally of obstetrical wit but in no time a twin girl was delivered. I must have been forgiven for my remark because I was made godfather to the girl.

"Next time, Kate," I told her later, "you jolly well come to the office at least once during your time. You did not know as much about it all as you thought."

"Maybe not," she replied, "but I still know a damn sight more about it all than you do." There was no point in denying the obvious.

The final tally of children eventually reached thirteen. Bill got confused over their names and ages and, according to Kate, was shamefully delinquent in attending to their needs, failing to help with them as a good father should. Once, when they travelled to America with a score then of about eleven, the airlines competed for their patronage, not because of the mass booking, but on account of their publicity value. On colour TV the swarm of redheads climbing the aircraft steps was worth a mint of advertising. It was on one of these flights, when Kate was coping with her brood, that she had the surprise of her life. Ryan was sitting somewhat apart but bouncing a baby on his knee. She had never seen this before and stared in disbelief at this show of fatherly interest. A keener glance revealed that the baby was not one of their own, but belonged to the woman in the next seat.

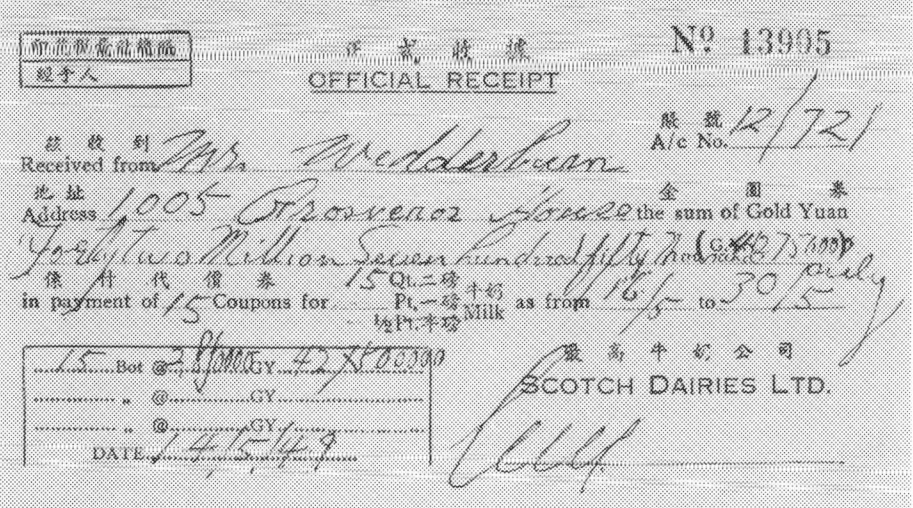

Milk receipt for forty-two million Gold Yuan.

Saw Battle From Air

Dr. R. G. W. Wedderburn, of Shanghai who was flown to Nanking on Wednesday in order to lend a hand if the casualties should be taken there told the "North-China Daily News" that he had witnessed part of the battle from the air. He saw spouts of water shooting up all around Consort, he said, and also saw puffs of smoke as her guns replied and the explosions when the shells landed.

Dr. Wedderburn returned from Nanking by train and assisted in the treatment of the wounded at the Country Hospital all day yesterday.

A young seaman from the Consort also gave the "North-China Daily News" a graphic description of the fight. He said that the ship sailed up and down sometimes as near as five hundred yards from the north bank "We were firing point blank over open sights for most of the time," he said.

Nine Guns Knocked Out

He said that they knocked out at least nine communist gun emplacements.

This man also said that the communist seemed to have five-inch guns in action.

They came very near to passing a tow to Amethyst according to his account but she signalled them to stand clear and avoid danger. They were being fired on by then and the captain of the Consort decided to steam straight on and turn round to make another attempt from downstream. On the second run past the batteries they suffered all the casualties.

Four or five holes were visible on the starboard side of Consort. Two had been plugged and two patched overnight.

The Consort and the Amethyst are both light escort vessels which carry no armour and are not designed for battle engagements but for anti-submarine and anti-aircraft protection, a naval officer told this paper.

From the North China Daily News.

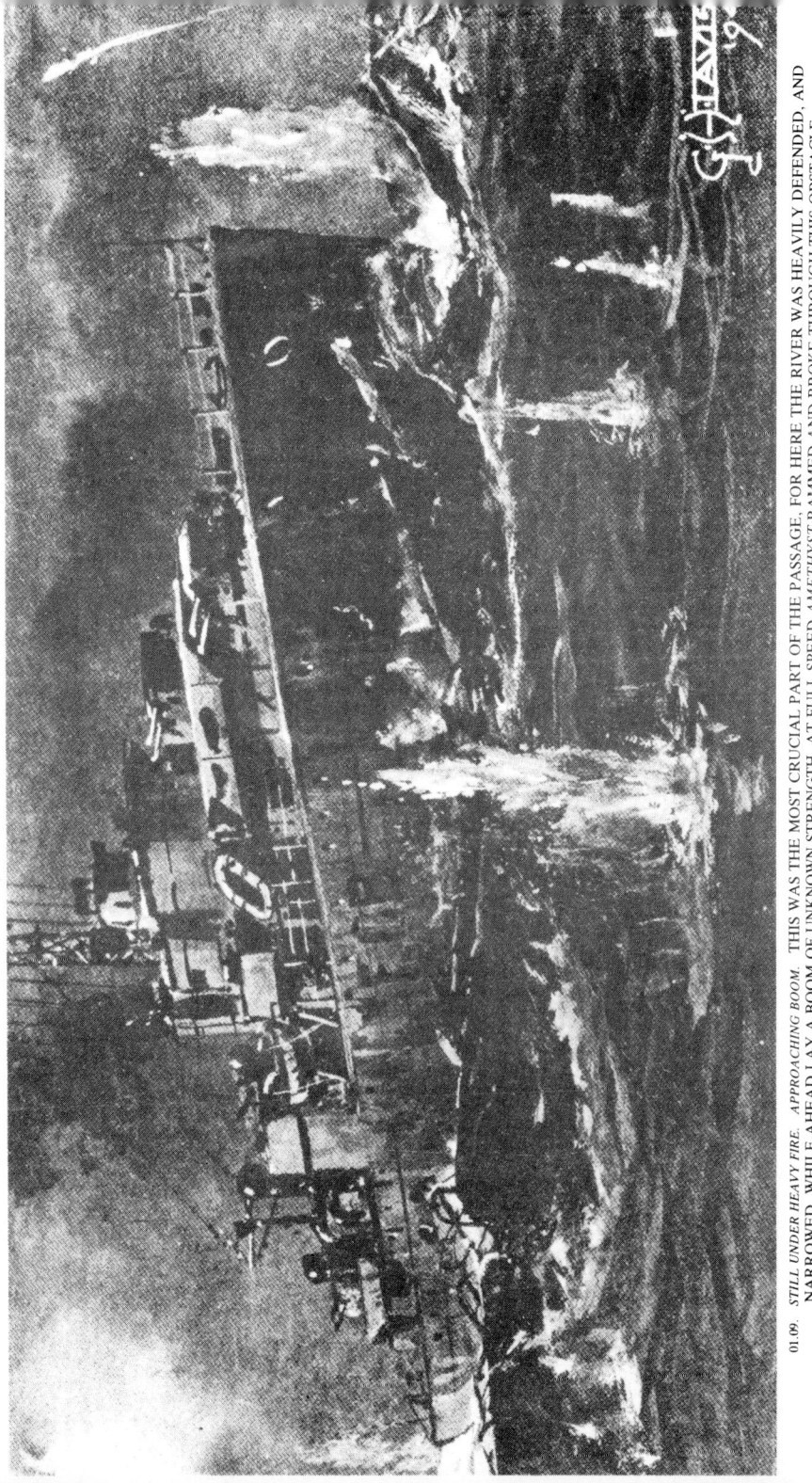

01.09. *STILL UNDER HEAVY FIRE. APPROACHING BOOM.* THIS WAS THE MOST CRUCIAL PART OF THE PASSAGE, FOR HERE THE RIVER WAS HEAVILY DEFENDED, AND NARROWED, WHILE AHEAD LAY A BOOM OF UNKNOWN STRENGTH. AT FULL SPEED *AMETHYST* RAMMED AND BROKE THROUGH THIS OBSTACLE.

From the Illustrated London News.

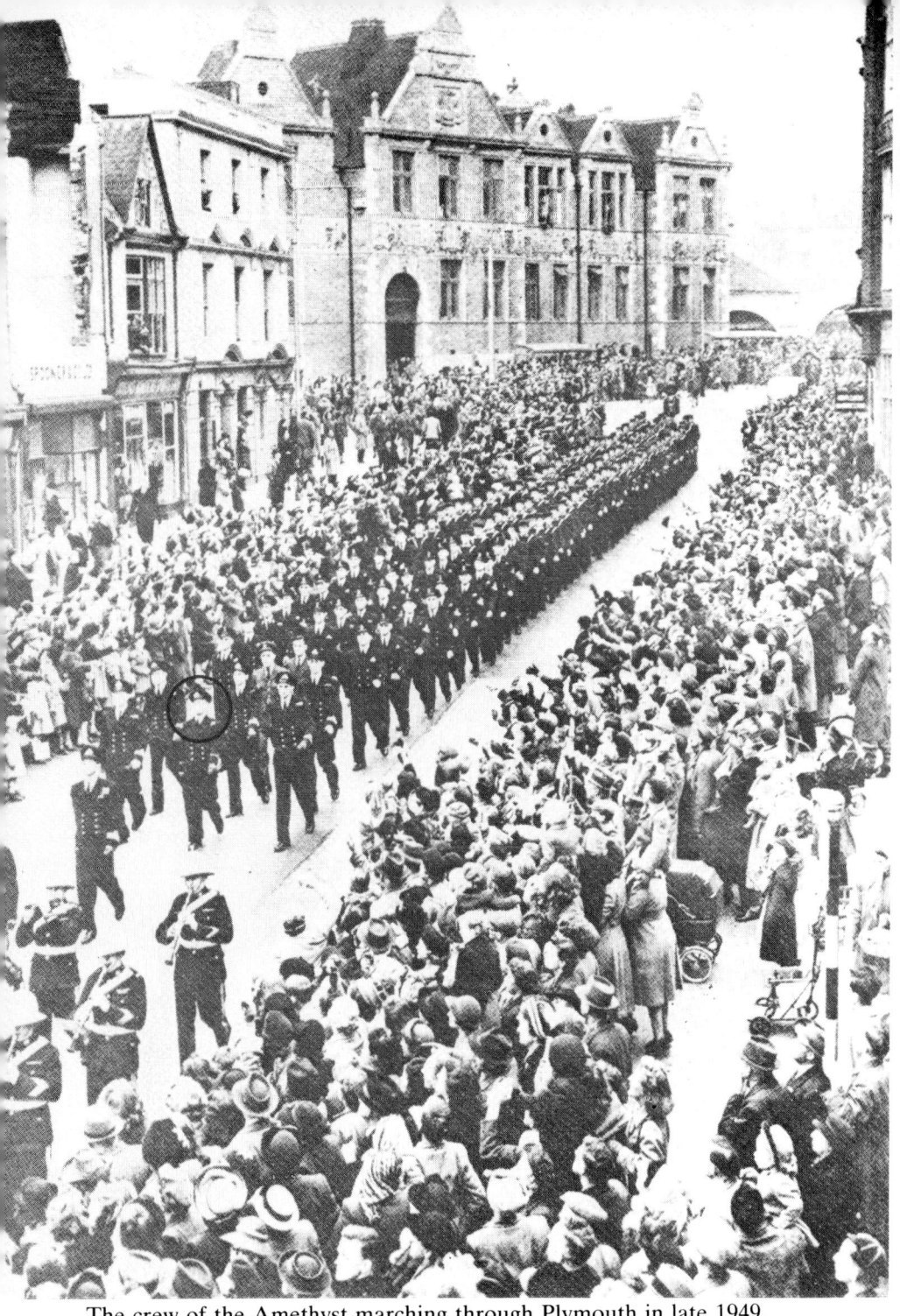

The crew of the Amethyst marching through Plymouth in late 1949.

Lt. Weston is circled.

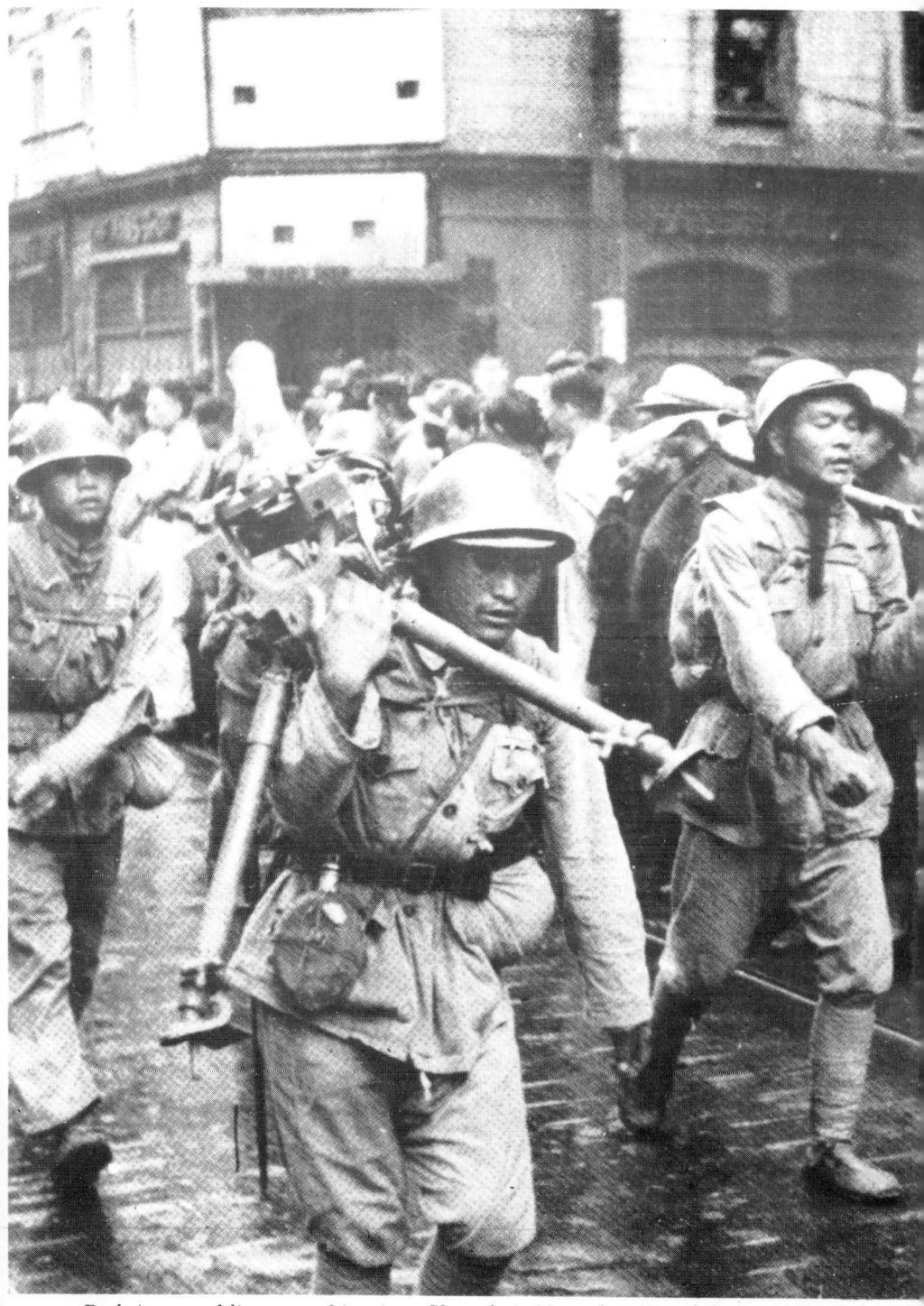

Red Army soldiers marching into Shanghai. Note the size of the machine-gun.

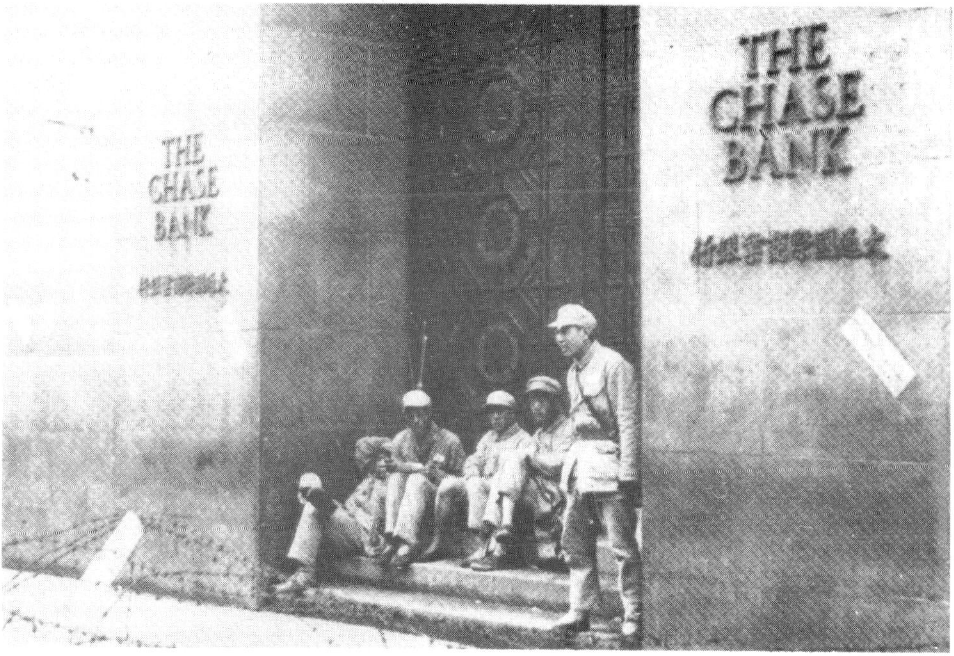

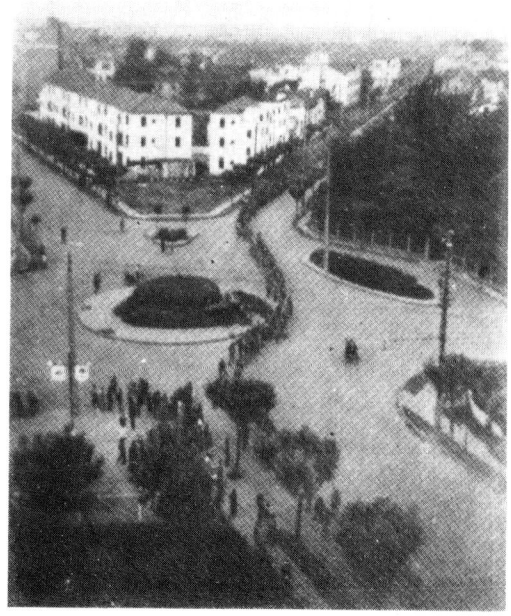

(Above) *Even conquerors must rest.*
(Right) The Red Army marched
into Shanghai in the early hours of
May 23, 1949. The photograph was
taken from the penthouse of
Cavendish Court, Avenue Petain.

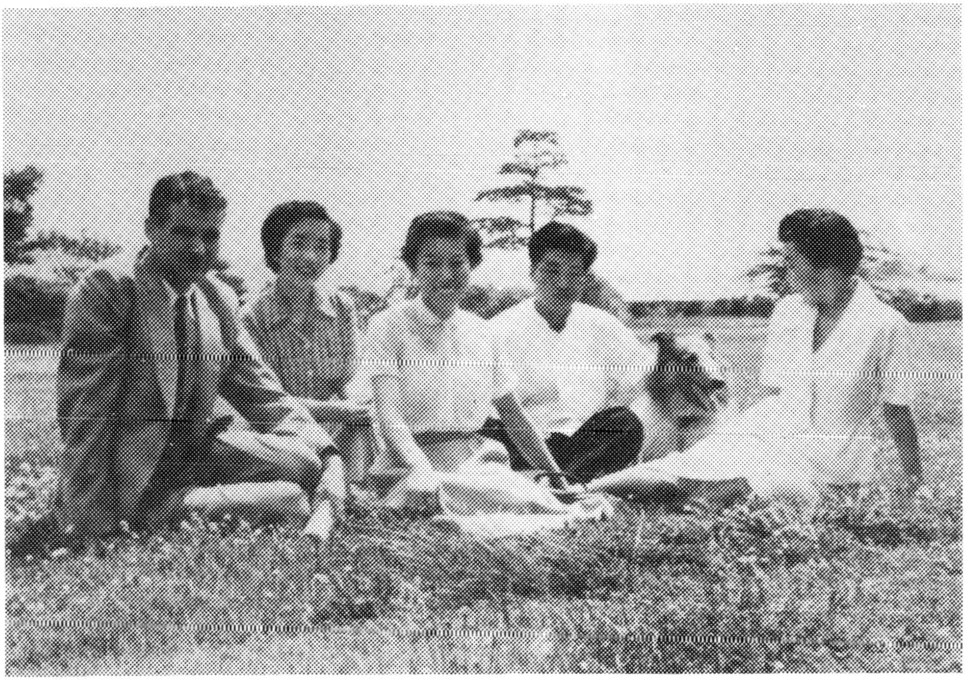

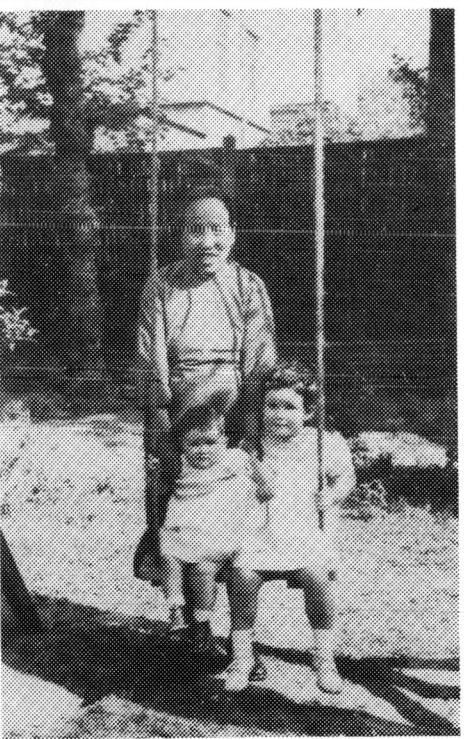

(Above) *With staff from the clinic.*
(Left) *At River House in 1950. Siu Ying came with us for the first year in Japan.*

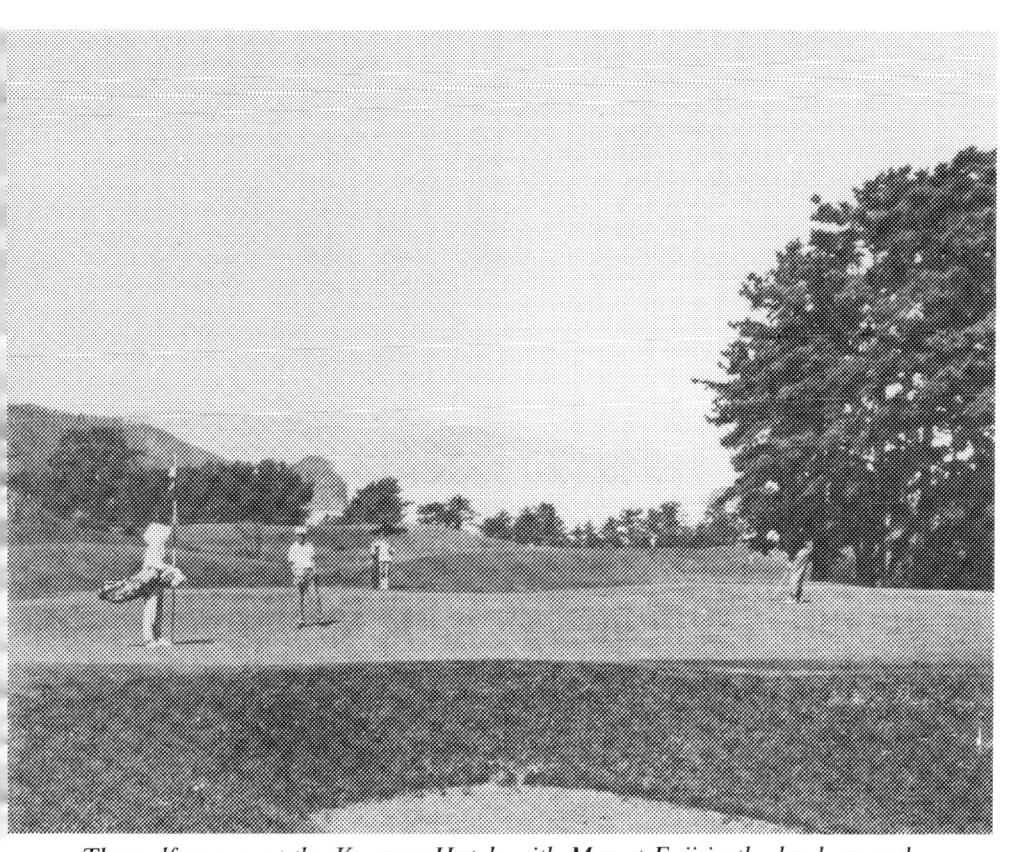

The golf-course at the Kawana Hotel, with Mount Fuji in the background.

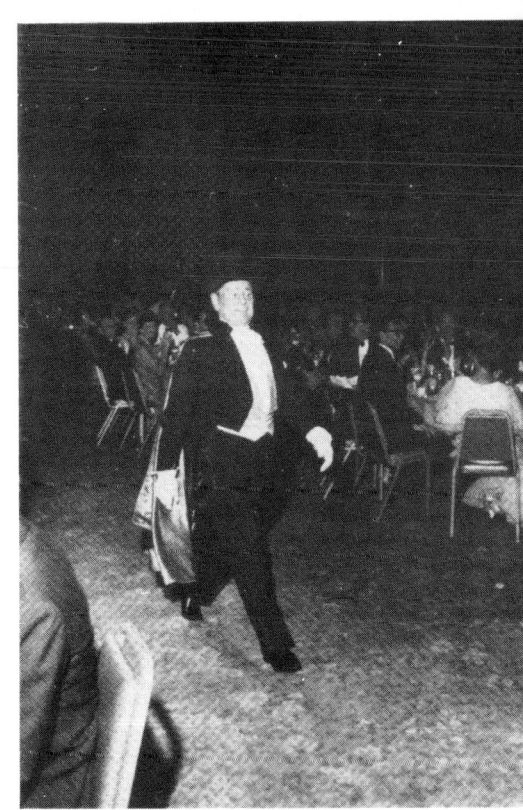

(Right) *John Besford, President of the Loyal Ball in 1969, during the visit of Princess Margaret.* (Below) *John Besford's house at Aberatsubo.*

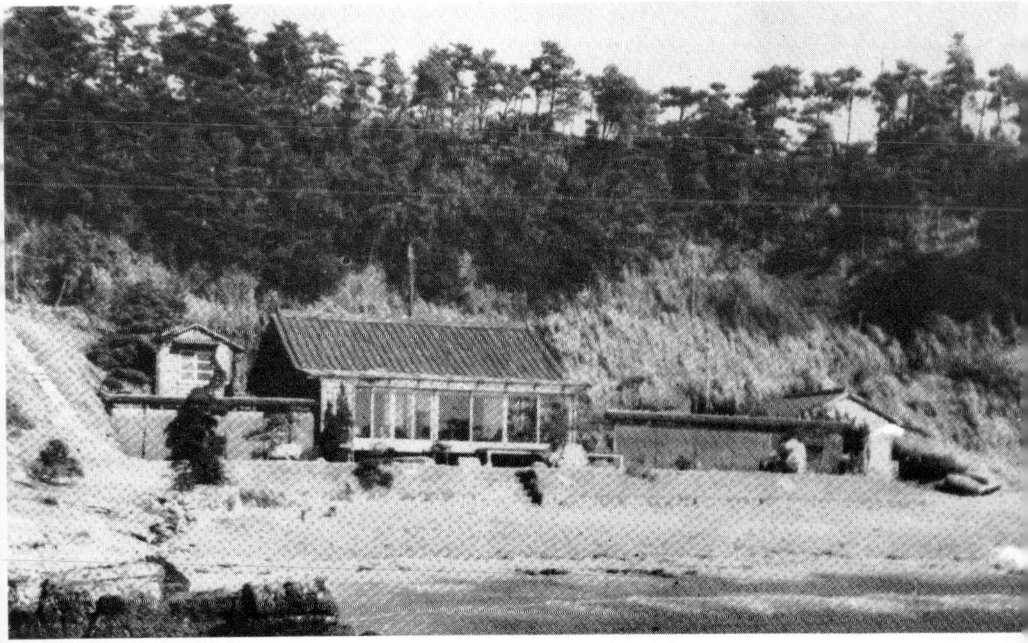

"What the hell are you doing, Ryan?" she asked. "What about ours?"

"Kate, dear, you know all about looking after children. This poor woman has just had her first and is quite inexperienced."

At the time that the Ryans lived next door, the yard which separated the two houses was part of their lease; our house had a small garden in front. On most days the yard was full of lines supporting a mass of children's garments and nappies hung out to dry. There was obviously a great deal of washing being done and it annoyed Jean and myself to find out that the Ryans' monthly water bill was in the region of one thousand yen, whereas ours was between three and four thousand. Furthermore, a man nearby, who had a small swimming pool, filled it once a week from the mains supply, not bothering with a filter or other mechanical device. Having pulled the plug out and emptied and cleaned the pool, he turned the tap on at bedtime leaving the water to run in all night, and by morning the pool was nearly full. Despite this extravagance, his water bill in summer was less than ours. We asked the water authorities to investigate. A man inspected our house and pointed out that the tap to the bath leaked and dripped. The plug was put in and by morning there was less than an inch of water in the bath. When the inspector returned at my request, he made no comment. I took him into the yard and showed him the Ryans' laundry lines. On that day they had surpassed themselves. I do not think I have ever seen such a massive display of garments hung out to dry.

I told him, "There you are, there are ten in that family plus the maids. They are Americans. Apart from the washing, Americans, as you know, are always taking showers every hour of the day. How is it that their bill is one quarter of ours?" There was no explanation, but if we did not pay, the supply would be cut off. It was the principle of the matter which irritated me.

In winter, drying clothes in the damp Tokyo air is a long and unsatisfactory process, so I was persuaded to buy an electric dryer. Nothing in Japan was that easy. The dryer needed a special fifteen amp cable, a discovery made after its delivery.

The cable had to be run from the supply some seventy yards from the house. Needless to say, the cost of buying the cable and laying it underground was more than the dryer. A gang of three workmen arrived and started digging a trench across our garden.

It was typical of Tokyo that fairly decent houses and what were little better than shacks marched cheek by jowl. Across the lane which gave access to our compound was a small village of very poor quality houses crowded densely together.

"When anything happens," Jean telephoned me, "you are always out or in the office."

"What has happened?" I asked.

"The men laying the cable blocked off a pipe under the lawn and the complete water supply of the village has been interrupted. Absolute mayhem is reigning."

The pipe was connected to our meter.

This state of affairs was put right and the supply reinstated. The advice tendered by some of my friends to create merry hell with the water authority was not followed. There was a great deal of face lost all round which is a grievous thing in the Orient. It was much better to let the matter slide; it would have aggravated the loss of face to claim redress which would not in any event materialise. We awaited our next water bill with interest. It was one hundred and twenty yen and remained at this figure for six months after which time it gradually crept up to a normal one thousand. By various small manifestations, however, it became apparent that the people who lived across the lane became less friendly and bore us some animosity thereafter. They, too, had lost face. It was unlike the Japanese not to have solved the problem by giving us a big Christmas present or making some other small gesture of friendship, to be followed in its turn by some reciprocal gesture on our part. It was not for us, the wronged party, to make the first move.

Japanese gardens differ from all other gardens. Flowers as such play only a minor role. Paved paths wind around clumps of bushes and trees, and a pool, possibly crossed by a stone bridge or stepping stones, is usually a feature. Carved stone lanterns or the statue of a goddess stand to form a feature, but not a dominating one. There are a few flowers, but their presence is muted. Lawns are almost unknown. Until the advent of golf swept the land, there was little grass to be seen, with a corresponding lack of knowledge of its cultivation and care. Undeterred by the difficulties, a supplier was found who laid a lawn in the small garden which fronted our house to end against a six-foot wall separating the property from the lane beyond. The lawn looked great for about two weeks, but then started to deteriorate and eventually became a few irregular patches of tired-looking grass surrounded by patches of earth and pebbles. The lawn met its final demise with the arrival of the logs.

With our fireplace built and ready to heat the lounge as well as dissipate its warmth through the walls, some considerable quantity of fuel was a necessity. Over lunch a friend told me that he was ordering logs from Kariuzawa, the upland plateau where houses could be rented in summer to escape the heat and humidity of the Japanese summer. He had not finalised his order and if I wanted some logs he would order for me as well.

"How much are you getting?" I asked.

"Oh, a railway wagon load."

"Good," I said, "order me a wagon load too."

In due course the railway wagons arrived at Shibuya station and my friend arranged for the logs to be shipped by truck.

"Better be at home when they arrive," he said.

At the appointed hour three vast trucks pulled into the lane. Up to that time I had not visualised a railway wagon nor realised its capacity. Each truck had a driver with two workers who, without delay, started unloading over the wall into the garden. The logs were a fine grade of birch with a silver bark. Each log was cut to almost three foot lengths and they came over the wall in a cascade. The piles got bigger and bigger. Soon the garden was covered by a mass of logs, and still they came, bouncing over each other. I watched with trepidation as what must have been the tree population of a sizeable forest continued to accumulate, with the third truck still waiting to get alongside the wall. By the time the third truck had deposited its load the grass was completely hidden. Working in most of my spare time it took nearly a month for me to stack the logs in an orderly fashion along the wall of the lane and the bamboo fence of the driveway. The stacks reached a height of six feet, forming an impressive sight. Their sheer volume reduced the area of the garden considerably and the grass had taken a pounding from which it subsequently never recovered.

The bamboo fence on the opposite side of the garden from the driveway was reserved for the oil drums. In the constant battle to hold the seeping cold at bay we had installed two large oil space heaters, one in the hallway and the second in the children's playroom. Experience of the previous winter had shown that in order to feel secure, it was necessary to buy the oil in forty-five gallon drums sometime in September. The important consideration was to have enough of them. Around December there was an acute shortage of the drums themselves and since the only way to get replenishments was to offer two empty drums for a full one, we started the autumn with nine full drums. The presence of the drums along the east fence did nothing to enhance the aesthetic appearance of our garden, but with logs and oil in sufficient amounts, one was battened down for winter and ensured of at least keeping the chill off, if both fuels were used in the most profligate way. The oil space heaters were turned on full blast, and logs were hurled on the fire recklessly. When it got really cold in January and February, an occasional gas fire or electric heater contributed its quota of heat.

The logs from Kariuzawa were green and for the first few weeks coal was needed to keep them going. There were logs on the fire and others around it drying out. Sap oozed out of the ends of the logs. They hissed, cracked and sometimes banged like a pistol shot. Jean gloomily predicted that this would go on all winter but curiously the birch dried out very quickly. After six weeks the fires would keep going without coal, and by Christmas coal was not necessary even at the lighting of the fire. By the following autumn there was a reserve of dried logs still remaining and my friend and I shared a railway wagon load each subsequent winter.

While the husband of the family concerned himself with the long term mechanical improvements and gasped with amazement at the financial estimates for them, the housewife struggled on with the day-to-day complexities of living, baffled from time to time by events which were completely unpredictable. Jean found a carpenter to make a table and two small chairs for our girls to eat at in the children's room. The girls were more or less measured by the carpenter for the size of the chairs and table height. He departed with his measurements and in a week returned to exhibit proudly *one* chair and *two* tables. I do not think Jean ever fully recovered from the blow.

Only once again was she so completely perplexed. As we prepared to leave Japan, she handed in our resident cards. Consternation was registered by the emigration authorities and an impasse reached. While hers, mine and the elder two girls' entry visas were in order, Victoria, our youngest, then age two, had no entry visa to Japan. Why? Because she had been born in Japan and, although the birth certificate stated this quite clearly, the official could think of no way of circumventing the regulation. One is at a loss to explain this discrepancy; it is not as though Victoria was unique. We had only to think of the Ryans next door who had perpetrated this misdemeanour several times without apparent let or hindrance, and departed in a blaze of publicity short of a lot of entry visas.

Chapter 21

THE CONSUL

The troublesome male witch — A difference in attitudes — Coming to the aid of young love.

The outbreak of a war or pestilence on a large scale anywhere at the present time would inevitably find nationals of almost every country in the globe involved. With cheap jet travel people swarm all over the world, but pre-war Japan was about as far flung from Britain as anywhere. Getting there involved a long expensive voyage and the land was alien. Foreigners were subject to ostracism and near persecution from the *Kenpeitai*, the secret police. Yet there was an extraordinary number of British in Japan, excluding businessmen, diplomats and the like. The British, who wanted to be there and had made up their minds to stay, come what may, were there. The occasional language professor and his wife, artists, eccentrics and a few women who had married Japanese remained in Japan. After the war most of these people had fallen on hard times and with advancing years many were living in abject poverty.

Sooner or later some agency, charitable or missionary, would become involved with their plight and when this happened it was inevitable that somewhere along the line a doctor would be called in. As the only British doctor in Japan, that meant me. The approach to me was invariably made on grounds of nationality and compassion; my efforts were very unrewarding. Firstly, for a variety of obscure reasons, these people would never come to see me, so I had to go to them; secondly, what was offered was not what they wanted. Basically, they wanted better housing and living conditions, with sufficient financial support to continue to stay exactly where they were, but the charitable organisations usually thought that repatriation to the United Kingdom was what was needed. The many bottles of vitamin pills, tins of powdered milk or canned vegetables which accrued from my visits were stacked in the storeroom and just took up space. The unwilling supplicants did not even have the gumption to sell these gifts for profit.

The British Embassy knew all about these people and their recalcitrant attitudes and would make a determined attempt to help them but, after several attempts and rebuffs, the Embassy accepted the status quo and kept their names on file against the time when they would become infirm and helpless. It fell to the lot of the British Consul, Leo Pickles, to deal with them when that time came.

Leo Pickles was typical of the best of our consuls. A British consul, if he is worth his salt, and most of them are, goes into action almost automatically in support of one of his nationals, right or wrong. One day, he came into my office, sat down and started on the story of one such unfortunate British subject. He was surprised by my lack of resistance to the plea for help, but Pickles was not one who asked often or without good cause. His honesty was apparent, and his very diffidence commanded respect.

Mrs Nakayama was such a case. She was a Japanese national but ethnically English. She had married a Japanese before the war, was in Japan during the war, and was now a widow. She was destitute and subsisted on the little money that her son, who had a very poorly paid job in Tokyo, managed to give her. The son had approached the Embassy as his mother had been English. Pickles explained that this presented a peculiar problem as there were no funds or official channels to deal with such a person who was technically a Japanese. Nevertheless, he hoped to help her and, though it was not my line of country as she was mentally abnormal, a case for repatriation might be made out for her if a medical report was pitched in strong enough terms. She lived in the country and the best part of a day would be needed for a visit for which my only reward would be his thanks.

It was a cold dark morning when an Embassy car called for me. The driver set off through the incredibly drab northern section of Tokyo and out into the Kanto plain. The small villages we passed were depressing. The country, broken up into small fields, was bleak in the February morning. The roads were of gravel and narrow, and seemed to intersect aimlessly. Progress was slow and far from comfortable. At times, the car pulled half off the road, close to ditches full of evil-looking water, to allow other vehicles to pass. Flurries of sleet beat on the windows of the car. As we cleared the town the driver handed me a note from Pickles. Presumably he had been told to hold on to it until the signs of civilisation had fallen behind and I could not change my mind.

I opened it and read.

"Dear Dr Wedderburn,

When you meet Mrs Nakayama it would be better not to

mention that you are a doctor or a Scot. Avoid the subject of politics. Perhaps it would be best if you said you were a member of the Embassy.

She is troubled by a witch.

Regards,
L. Pickles."

I looked for a second page in explanation of these cryptic warnings but there was nothing else in the envelope. By now it had started snowing in earnest. A cup of coffee in some congenial inn would have made a welcome halt but nothing that looked remotely like a suitable place came into view. In the late morning we drew up at a small hamlet at a crossroads. The driver indicated that we were at our destination.

Squelching through some mud I pulled aside the *shoji* door, took my shoes off and entered, immediately realising that the temperature inside was no warmer than out, and that my thin socks were not going to preserve my feet in any degree of comfort. Mrs Nakayama greeted me in Japanese but soon got the hang of the fact that English was my preferred medium. She was tallish, gaunt, and with long, dark grey unkempt hair. Sombre eyes stared at me. Her dress was black and hung in uneven folds. She was not quite one of the witches in Macbeth but going on that way.

We crouched cross-legged on the *tatami* floor at a low table with nothing to support our backs. I kept my overcoat and gloves on but my toes were already icy. A small bowl of tepid Japanese tea did not match my thoughts of hot coffee.

We chatted away for a quarter of an hour about where she came from in England, her son in Tokyo, the countryside, the weather and so on. She seemed normal enough and even rose in my estimation for a few seconds when she asked me what position I held in the Embassy.

This caught me short for a moment before I vouchsafed that I was Head of Chancery. It was the first idea which occurred to me and seemed a likely enough post. There was some justification for this assumption as a short while previously I had extracted half the stomach and the first part of the duodenum from the Head of the Chancery; this action for his duodenal ulcer gave me some ephemeral rights for such a claim, I felt.

"Oh," said Mrs Nakayama, disappointed. "I thought you were the Ambassador!"

162

Seldom has a simple surgeon set off in the morning as a plain citizen, been accepted into the Diplomatic Corps by late breakfast time, promoted afterwards to Head of the Chancery, to become obvious ambassadorial material by coffee-break time.

As all feeling had now long since gone from my feet and the frost-bite was about mid-calf level, I decided to hurry things along. I was well aware that a psychiatrist would have approached the problem in an oblique fashion. Mrs Nakayama's childhood, relations with her mother and father, relations with her boyfriends, dreams, feelings, psyche and conscious elements would have been established as a base before the present was tactfully introduced. Aware of my lack of knowledge on these matters, I adopted as an alternative the plain, brusque, direct, surgical approach.

"I understand, Mrs Nakayama," I said, "that you are troubled by a witch."

The floodgates were opened. It was long and complicated but in essence this was the story.

There was; she said, a Scots doctor who practised in Harley Street in London. The doctor had a witch at his disposal, and a very degenerate and willing tool the witch was. From time to time the Prime Minister would visit the doctor and ask him to despatch the witch to Japan to trouble Mrs Nakayama. The Scots doctor, a really rotten type, was only too happy to oblige the Prime Minister, and off the witch went without delay. That was bad enough, but the Scots doctor took a malicious pleasure in this activity and, working entirely on his own initiative, would send off the witch unknown to the Prime Minister, the Foreign Office, the Secret Service or any other Government agency. The Prime Minister had a lot of problems on his hands. This action was a sort of mental aberration on his part, not to be condoned of course, but politicians were, after all, politicians. The Prime Minister requested the doctor to provide this service about once a year but the doctor took it upon himself to make this a monthly occurrence. There was only one slight saving grace: the Prime Minister might want the witch for other nefarious tasks, so that about four days was as long as he could be absent without the Scots doctor having to answer embarrassing questions.

The warnings in Pickles' note were now amply clear. Having kept quiet about being Scots and a doctor, I hastened to assure Mrs Nakayama that it was my impression that the diplomatic corps were not allowed to vote politically, and secondly, that I had never been in

Britain during an election, had never voted and, furthermore, had never lost a wink of sleep at being deprived of the privilege. I was glad to be able to make three truthful statements in a row.

The witch, it transpired, was not of the female sex. He was a very nasty little man standing four feet high. He wore a long dark green cloak to keep him warm, pretty sensible it would seem in view of the heating problem in the Nakayama household. When he travelled he spread this cloak as wings, no broom or other aid to aviation forming part of his equipment. He made the journey London-Tokyo in four hours flat.

"What does the witch do that upsets you?" I asked Mrs Nakayama.

It was his presence, rather than anything else, that upset her, she answered. He was always in the room with her, and it was very embarrassing when she wanted to undress and go to bed. He bothered her. She was shocked when my enquiries indicated that the witch might have taken liberties. As an amateur psychiatrist, I felt that Freud and sexual questions should somehow be brought into the matter. No, there was no question of that sort of thing. She was not frightened, just bothered. The witch dossed down in the corner of the bedroom and she would finally go off to sleep, only to wake and find him still there. He never spoke and suddenly, after a few days, he would go without farewell or salutation.

"When was he last here?" I asked.

"Over three weeks ago."

"You mean he may be back any time?"

"Yes."

I took a quick peek over my shoulder just in case he had arrived ahead of schedule. I felt the facts were marshalled, and it was time I was gone.

I only saw Mrs Nakayama once more after that, when my nurse came with me to the Embassy to give Mrs Nakayama her cholera and smallpox innoculation immediately prior to her departure. When Pickles asked me why it was necessary for the nurse to be there I enjoyed watching his eyebrows shoot up half an inch on being told that Mrs Nakayama would think it strange to have the Head of Chancery sticking needles into her.

The case of Jimmy Baekker illustrates the quality of a man like Leo Pickles, who would extend his courtesy to any national, British or otherwise. Jimmy, an American businessman with an office down the corridor from ours, was picked up by the police for a currency offence. One of the dollar cheques he had passed for yen turned up in Kobe, and Jimmy was taken off to jail. He languished for six weeks in Kobe jail.

"The Japanese have not heard of Habeas Corpus. They don't understand Latin," he told me in explanation of the length of his incarceration.

The first thing he did on being established as an inmate was to ask the American consul to see him. The consul turned up, listened to Jimmy's story, read Jimmy a lecture on breaking the law of Japan, told him that he must bear the consequences of his misdemeanours and walked out. The door was slammed, followed by the sound of bolts being rammed home and the prisoner was left alone and forlorn.

Jimmy was not without resource, and relations with his captors were soon cordial. Minor breaches of regulations occurred, such as the sharing out to the police of the cigarettes and liquor he purchased. After five days Jimmy was allowed to stay in a hotel and report to the police station twice daily. Some more chocolates and whisky reduced this to a once daily ritual, but stay in Kobe he did.

As he had a lot of time to ponder, he devoted much of it to thinking about his consul and his conclusions were not flattering. Jimmy was on his own and a drawn-out legal battle followed. He took me through his ordeal step by step after his return to his Tokyo haunts. Very soon afterwards, a British businessman was arrested on the same charge, on the afternoon of his planned departure by BOAC at 9.30 p.m. Pickles was in action straightaway with a visit to the prisoner and a quick call at the Foreign Office. Intensive negotiations followed which resulted in a bond of surety being lodged. Pickles himself attended the man's release.

"I am sorry," apologised Pickles. "You missed the BOAC flight, but I have booked you on Pan Am at eleven. If we hurry we can just make it."

When this story came to my ears and I related it to Jimmy he started talking wildly about dashing off to the British Consulate to change his nationality. I was able to persuade him that this was not a sufficient reason to give up his birthright.

"After all," I said, "you were both guilty."

Pickles became a good friend of my partner, Bernard Rosenberg, and his wife Susan. Eventually he became involved in a problem concerning their daughter.

Evelyn, the daughter, was an attractive and talented girl. Educated first at the French School in Shanghai and then at the American School in Tokyo and speaking German at home, she was truly trilingual.

After leaving school Evelyn went to the Interpreter's School in Geneva. Pupils have to be very gifted in languages to be accepted, and must become completely bilingual, preferably with a wide knowledge not only of a language but also of its literature, so that a quotation from the classics can be simultaneously matched by a similar quotation in the other tongue, plucked from the translator's mind. The best pupils and the most highly paid go on to work at international conferences, the United Nations and the like.

The Master of the School told her parents that because Evelyn only spoke German at home and had not been taught German literature in the manner in which she had been taught French and English literature at school, German, although her mother tongue, was in fact her poorest language. She could act as a simultaneous translator in English and French but would find it more difficult to work in German.

Bernard and Susan saw a brilliant future for their daughter, possibly culminating in a marriage to a European, moving from capital city to capital city in an aura of sophistication and culture. It therefore came like a clap of thunder when Evelyn, then in her second year at Geneva, wrote to say that she had decided to give up the course and get married.

Bernard explained this to me.

"And," he said, "she wants to marry an Englishman, so bourgeois." He hesitated, realising that he might have hurt my feelings.

I well realised that he was making the mistake so commonly made by foreigners of lumping together all the inhabitants of Britain as Englishmen, and in other circumstances might have remonstrated. However, he was so obviously upset that I let him off the hook.

"Dear Bernard," I said, "We Scots consider the English to be much inferior to ourselves."

Every effort was made to dissuade Evelyn, or at least get her to complete the course in Geneva. When all else had failed, Susan Rosenberg got hold of information which led her to believe that there might be a regulation in British law which might at least put a damper on an alien under twenty-one marrying a citizen of the United Kingdom, and she resolved to ask for an appointment with Leo Pickles to seek help and clarification. Pickles knew the Rosenbergs well, and there is little doubt that he was aware, at least vaguely if not accurately, of the reason for the interview.

Mrs Rosenberg duly presented herself in his office. They drank tea, looked out on the lawn of the Embassy, and discussed various trivialities until Pickles asked what he could do for her.

"Well," she said, "you know Evelyn is German and is only nineteen and she wants to marry an Englishman."

Pickles was sympathetic, would have wanted to help, but he was still Her Britannic Majesty's Consul General in Japan. His deep, slow, sonorous voice was hauled up, not from his chest, but from his very boots.

"Seems to me," he paused for reflection, "to be a very, very good idea!"

In the end she did marry her Englishman and went to live near Manchester, brought up a family and was totally happy with her lot.

Chapter 22

A SEA VOYAGE AND SUNKEN TREASURE

Skirting a typhoon — Shipboard party — The furniture goes overboard.

When Jean and the girls were due back by ship in Hong Kong, I decided to go there to meet them. With Derek and Bernard, the clinic had then been running for over a year. During the first year, whenever I managed to get away early from the hospital I could always see someone in downtown Tokyo on some relevant business matter. One morning, having done my round of the patients, there was some time to spare, and I suddenly realised that there was no one or no matter concerning either my own or the clinic's affairs to visit. It was the "end of the beginning". The clinic was set up and set fair.

Deciding that I had been working hard without let up for a long time, a sea voyage seemed to be a good idea. A leisurely four days on a freighter to Hong Kong would be ideal. There was a Norwegian ship, the *Temeraire* of the Barber Wilhelmsen Line, leaving from Kobe. Having arrived in Kobe, I put my gear on board, noticing the blackboard at the top of the gangway which notified crew and passengers that the ship would sail next morning at 7.00 a.m. Owing to the attentions of my friends in Kobe I embarked at 5.00 a.m. and watched my friends depart along the dock. Breakfast passed without my presence. An elderly stewardess gave me coffee before I started to find the whereabouts of the decks, lounge, and dining saloon. There were no other passengers, the lounge was full of heavy Norwegian pine furniture, and the library held only Norwegian books. The desired restful sea voyage was obviously going to be very restful indeed.

Only the Captain dined in the passenger saloon My place was laid at the opposite end of a long table. Captain Vasser was finishing his lunch when we introduced ourselves and it was not until dinner that we had an opportunity for conversation. I was a bit surprised when Captain Vasser drank a glass of beer and then an aquavit without offering me any such refreshment. Not until lunch the following day did it transpire that the MV *Temeraire* had been on the

New York-Lagos-West Africa run for a few years and the only passengers she had carried had been missionaries, all of whom had been very strictly teetotal. Captain Vasser assumed that I was one also; meals were staid affairs until the misconception was cleared up. He told me that he always played the mouth-organ accompaniment for the hymns sung on Sundays at the services held by the missionaries. He produced one from a drawer in the table and rendered "Onward Christian Soldiers".

I helped myself to another aquavit.

They could only have three hymns, "Onward Christian Soldiers" and two others, as those completed the Captain's whole repertoire.

As the strains of music faded, a message was given to the Captain. "There is a typhoon south of us. Excuse me, please," he said before leaving for the bridge.

He was back shortly to tell me that he had altered course due East to avoid the expected track of the typhoon and consequently our trip would last at least five days instead of four. We went up to the bridge to look at the typhoon maps. As it was October, the tracks of all the October typhoons for the previous twenty years had been put on the chart. Red lines started to the east of the Philippines, some ran across the Philippine Islands across the Gulf of Thailand and into Vietnam; others went further north to hit the coast near Hainan Island and the south coast of China. Some lines skirted Taiwan, moved up past Okinawa and Japan, others bent north more rapidly, turned out into the Pacific and ended in indeterminate dots near the Aleutians. The present one was curving rapidly into the Pacific and heading towards the position of the *Temeraire* which Captain Vasser marked X on the chart with a bold stroke of his pen.

Next morning we looked at the chart again. Typhoon Ida had curved further into the Pacific. The estimated track now curved further east, passing through another X marking our new position.

"What are you going to do, Captain?"

"Keep going due east on our present course," said Captain Vasser.

"Look at this one," I said. "It did a circle out here off the Ryukyus." My finger followed the line to its origin.

"That one was in 1938," was the response.

"OK, Captain, but how long will the voyage take now?"

"At least six days."

Typhoon Ida, typically female, changed her mind to head due

169

north so that *Temeraire* would be influenced only by the remote edges of her vicious anti-clockwise movement. As we altered course due south, our plot still did not aim for Hong Kong but at least we were veering in the right direction. Our voyage time was now an estimated seven days. The weather on the margins of the typhoon was rough, sitting on deck was unpleasant, and I had long since thumbed through the few books in the lounge with pictures of fiords, mountains and Norwegian cows. My desired rest was far too restful, and frankly I was bored.

Six days out of Kobe the weather finally calmed down to a millpond smoothness and the ship's officers relaxed after playing hide and seek with the typhoon.

"I am afraid you have had rather a boring voyage," said Captain Vasser. "I tell you, I ask the Chief Officer and Chief Engineer, we have some drinks on deck and have dinner together. We have a little party. *Ja?*"

The ship would supply beer, aquavit and wine, and I would stand the after dinner drinks. Running the elderly stewardess to earth in her lair below decks I purchased the ship's total supply of Scotch, two bottles of John Haig Gold Label.

We met on deck at dusk. The ship was in the charge of the Second Mate. We had passed the southern tip of Taiwan on a direct course across the Taiwan Straits for Hong Kong. The sea was like a millpond bathed in the brilliant light of a tropical full moon.

We gripped our beer glasses and said "Skål".

We had an aquavit and said "Skål".

We held up our beer glasses and said "Cheers".

We had an aquavit and said "Cheers".

After this sally into English we confined ourselves to the Norwegian toast. Skål is such a satisfactory, crisp, appropriate word.

A few "Skåls" later we went into dinner with a couple of bottles of hock.

Back on deck it was my turn to be host. After the first empty bottle of Haig was cast overside, the Chief Officer in his rich sing-song Norwegian-accented English commented on the furniture in the passenger lounge.

"It is bloody awful, I think," he said.

"Oh, it is not too bad," I replied, mindful of the need to maintain Norwegian-Scottish relations.

"What do you think, Captain?" asked the First Mate.

"It is bloody awful, *ja?*" said the Captain.

"What do you think, Chief?" he asked the Engineer.

"It is bloody awful," replied the Engineer.

"What do you think now, doctor?"

"It is bloody awful," I replied.

"Well, let's throw it overboard," suggested the First Mate.

"*Ja,*" said the Engineer, a man of few words.

"Into the vater with it all," shouted the First Mate.

The tables and upright chairs presented no difficulty, and went over the rail with ease. The huge padded armchairs were more of a problem but by combined effort we got them out of the door and over the rail.

"*For et plask,*" yelled the Engineer. "What a splash."

The bookcase had been screwed to the wall by some stout Norwegian carpenter, and could not be prised loose.

Only the massive couch remained. We girded our loins.

"*Loft,*" ordered Captain Vasser. We attempted to lift it.

"*Det går ikke. Vi må dytte,*" advised the Chief Mate. It was no good, we must push.

"*Opp med'n,*" said the Captain and we heaved together.

"*Faen,*" shouted the Chief Engineer, as with a mighty ill-directed thrust we pinned him between the couch and a bulkhead. "*Faen*" means something like "goddammit", only stronger. We backed off, took a more accurate bearing on the door, upended it against the rail, strained, heaved, and got it balanced swinging seasaw on the rail. Slowly it toppled over, creating for long moments a huge hole in the moonlit waters of the South China Sea before it rapidly sank without trace.

Exhausted, we opened the second bottle and congratulated each other on a fine piece of teamwork.

The stewardess woke me with "*God morgen*" but she looked very disapproving indeed. I peered through the port-hole; we were anchored in Hong Kong harbour. Still disapproving, she helped me with my packing. I needed help. I went on deck making toward the bridge to say good-bye to Captain Vasser. I met him pacing slowly along the deck.

"How do you feel?" he asked.

"Bloody awful, thank you Captain. How about you?"

"Bloody awful, just like the furniture."

"By the way, Captain, you told me you were picking up five

passengers in Hong Kong. What will you do about furniture for the lounge?"

"Oh, the agents will buy some cheap rattan stuff here which will last till we get to Norway."

"It is already in the log. Damaged by bad typhoon weather," said Captain Vasser shaking me by the hand. "It was a good party, *ja?*"

I went down the gangway onto the motor launch and looked up at the Captain. He took a mouth organ from his pocket, leaned over the rail and started playing. I heard the first few bars of "Onward Christian Soldiers" before the launch turned away.

Fortunately, despite the delay I arrived in Hong Kong before my wife, Corinna and Alexi. We boarded a Glen Line vessel for a more conventional voyage to Yokohama, marked only by a slight difficulty at Customs in Japan. Jack McElney of Drs Anderson and Partners had sent on board a half carcass of a young sheep because I had mentioned to him that one could not buy lamb or mutton in Japan. A deep-frozen carcass baffled the Customs, but whether this was on account of import duty or a suspicion that a corpse was being disposed of never became clear.

The first letter I opened in my office on return contained a small memo sheet with the cryptic comment from a respected lawyer, "A sound investment. Recommend you purchase heavily."

The brochure with the memo contained the details relevent to the purchase of shares in the Pacific Far East Salvage Company Inc. The money, energies and endeavours of the company would be devoted entirely to the salvage of the cargo of the Russian Naval ship *Admiral Nakhimov* sunk by the Japanese halfway between Korea and Japan in the Tsashima Straits in 1905. She lay in 310 feet of water.

Her cargo consisted of 63 million gold sovereigns, worth then 630 million pounds sterling and now 2,640 million pounds or 5,000 million US dollars at the present day value.

I subscribed for shares immediately.

The Japanese attacked the Russian Forces in Manchuria in 1904, starting the Russo-Japanese war. As it progressed, Port Arthur on the tip of Manchuria's southern peninsula came under siege. Port Arthur was Russia's only warm water port in the East, indeed her only warm water port. To hold such a port was a Russian imperial dream; the dream to-day is no different.

To help to retain Port Arthur, the Tsar decided to send the

Russian Baltic Fleet all the way from Kronstadt through the Baltic, down the Atlantic to round the Cape of Good Hope, across the Indian Ocean, and up the China Sea to Port Arthur or Vladivostok.

Admiral Rozhdestvenski had his troubles. Three of the seven battleships were obsolete; there were five cruisers, nine torpedo boats and a hodge-podge of auxiliaries, not forgetting the *Kamchatka*, a repair ship. The *Kamchatka* spent most of her time calling on the other vessels to take on coal, and the crews were mostly land-based sailors of no experience. Gunnery training had been totally neglected and there was insufficient ammunition to allow either training or practice. The ships continually broke down. It says much for Rozhdestvenski that he brought the fleet into the Sea of Japan some nine months later in May 1905, having set sail in September 1904.

Why the good Admiral sailed his fleet between Japan and Korea remains a mystery, because Port Arthur had already fallen. He could have sailed well out in the Pacific, to turn to Vladivostok and there refurbish before offering battle.

Admiral Togo with his Japanese warships was waiting for the Russians in the Tsushima Straits where Togo promptly dealt with them, sinking eight major ships and capturing four. Of the entire fleet, only *Almoz*, formerly a steam yacht, and two destroyers limped into Vladivostock.

The *Admiral Nakhimov* was an armoured cruiser built in Glasgow on the River Clyde. The evidence of her cargo rests on the fact that while the Russian fleet sailed down the North Sea and English Channel they opened fire on some innocent English fishing trawlers in the belief that the Japanese had somehow sailed halfway round the world. There was talk of war between Britain and Russia, and the *Nakhimov*, which sailed into London, was understandably held up until tempers simmered down. While she was in the London river 63,000,000 gold sovereigns were withdrawn from the Bank of England by the Russian Embassy. The Embassy records were destroyed after the revolution.

The *Admiral Nakhimov*, tagging along in pursuit of the main body, arrived two days after the battle and was promptly despatched to the bottom of the Tsushima Straits. A few surviving sailors landed on Kyushu, the southern island of Japan, well equipped with gold sovereigns.

Salvage operations were conducted under the able direction of Mr Suzuki, aged then about 87, and he had been at the task on and off for twenty years. During World War II for instance, the Japanese navy recruited all Mr Suzuki's divers. The dives were "free dives". The diver wore a face mask connected to an air tube which delivered pumped air, but there was no sophisticated escape valve as the modern Scuba diving equipment. They could work only at that depth for three or four minutes to avoid the "bends" or Caisson disease. Diving could only be undertaken on clear, calm, sunny days for an hour on either side of noon.

Adequate funds were now available for Suzukisan to press ahead using an expanded diving force based on a more robust and seaworthy craft. The divers gradually cut their way through three decks using small explosive charges. Most of the ship had been searched, except for a few limited areas including the after gun turret and magazine. The fact that the after gun had not been fired during the action lent credence to the belief that the gold was stored either there or in the magazine. This belief, reasonable in most circumstances, could be open to a different interpretation if one studied the experiences and troubles of Admiral Rozhdestvenski. There may not have been sufficient gunners or ammunition; the officer with the key to the mechanism which turned the gun turret may have mislaid it or turret itself may have been faulty.

To confirm that Mr Suzuki and his lads had done what they claimed to have achieved, two divers from the US Navy were hired to have a look. They were very impressed indeed. Contrary to a commonly held impression, sea water preserves an iron or steel ship. It is exposure to air and oxygen after immersion which produces rapid damage. The divers went down on a good day when the water was clear. They reported the extraordinary sight of the ship apparently in perfect order resting on its keel on the seabed. Mr Suzuki's reports were accurate. The two divers were so favourably influenced by what they saw that they asked for only half of their fee if the other half was furnished in shares of the company.

About two years after the start of operations, I was elected to the board of directors. The third summer was unrewarding; bad weather limited diving and cash was running short, further aggravated by the loss of one of the divers whose family had to be compensated.

The board explored various possibilities in connection with the charter of a modern salvage vessel and several concerns showed interest, but such a venture was only feasible if there was a guaranteed worthwhile job in the Pacific somewhere near Japan. It would be a no cure — no pay affair with the salvage ship taking the lion's share. Lions can develop a rapacious appetite.

The possibility of putting a really sizeable charge against the after turret was discussed. The strategem was suggested by one member and had my support. As the only Scottish member of the board, this profligate scattering of sovereigns on the sea floor should have wrenched at my Scottish characteristics of thrift and frugality, but it was the Americans who demurred.

I brought the matter up at a subsequent meeting, to be stymied by the remark of the chairman, Tom van Nuys, who said, "Gren, you realise that *Admiral Nakhimov* was built in Glasgow and the armour plate — old boy — is Scottish steel. It would take a gigantic explosion to rip it apart."

This appeal to the patriotic pride I harboured in the good Scottish shipbuilders on the River Clyde was effective in deterring me from further endorsing the scheme. Secretly I still think we should have "had a go"; after all, what is the loss of two thousand million dollars if you win three thousand million?

The whole matter rests there and so does the *Admiral Nakhimov*.

When I left Japan, it was felt that for political reasons the secretary of the company might be better to be out of but near Japan, so in addition to remaining a director I also became secretary of the Pacific Far East Salvage Company Inc., opening a post-office box in Hong Kong so that I could read the numerous letters from anxious, hopeful, bewildered and sometimes angry shareholders. I forwarded the letters on to the chairman.

I am still the secretary today.

My original investment of US $200 has been well worth it. As a topic for dinner conversation, it fills the minds of my hosts with dreams extending beyond the natural bonds of human avarice. I have been plied with a myriad of glasses of expensive wines and fine old cognac as the guests come to realise that I control the possibility of their sharing in Eldorado, that some day I may be well Worth Knowing.

There the matter and the *Nakhimov* remained until the Chairman wrote to me from the USA in the early eighties that a Japanese businessman had organised a search with a modern vessel and equipment. Soon afterwards I heard again from the Chairman. Reports were circulating that the gold had been recovered. As a company we should take steps to ensure that our rights would not be usurped. Meanwhile, the Japanese government started to show considerable interest and the Russians got in on the act with a claim that the treasure was theirs.

The Chairman, Tommy van Nuys, was somewhat pessimistic regarding our chances of providing legal proof of our ownership. The company would have to engage lawyers in Japan at no mean expense and the Japanese Government formed a formidable opposition, not to mention the Russian claims.

The businessman held a press conference in Tokyo, a well attended conference. He displayed no gold but showed a large rectangular object weighing over 100 pounds which he claimed was platinum. Subsequently the heavy metal object proved to be a chunk of lead. My planned visit to the Rolls-Royce showroom was indefinitely postponed.

The passenger vessel "Admiral Nakhimov" was sunk in a collision in the Black Sea in 1986 with the loss of over 300 lives. The choice of this name for a liner or a warship must now be deemed to be unfortunate by the Russian authorities.

Chapter 23

THE GENERAL AND HIS SECRETARY

Grandpa and the railways — MacArthur's farewell — The little policeman who stole the show.

Bill Bloom was secretary to General Douglas MacArthur from the time that MacArthur became Supreme Commander; he sat in on all the conferences held by his chief both before and during the Korean War. He could take shorthand at a conference of six or seven men lasting an hour, and produce a typewritten transcript of every word said within an hour and a half. I watched him one evening take down some business letters from Bill Ryan, our next door neighbour, on a shorthand machine. Kate and I sat in the room interjecting comments and sometimes talking to each other. The session of dictation lasted forty minutes and in three quarters of an hour he produced the letters and a separate sheet with all the remarks made by Kate and myself. He did ask us to clear out of the room while he was doing the transcript.

Like all good secretaries Bill was the soul of discretion, and never spoke about what he heard. After MacArthur was dismissed, Bill continued as secretary, first to General Ridgway and then to General Mark Clark, who was the last overall Commander of the Allied Forces during the Korean War. I once asked Bill which he preferred.

"I like all three," he said. "I preferred working for MacArthur on Mondays and Thursdays, Ridgway on Tuesdays and Fridays, Mark Clark on Wednesdays and Saturdays." His ugly face creased with a charming smile.

"Sorry I asked, Bill," I replied.

Bill was a Catholic and had a large family of some seven or eight children. His wife's father, a widower, also lived with them. He was just known as Grandpa. Grandpa had worked all his life on the Santa Fe Railroad and somewhere along the line his memory had gone. Grandpa was a friendly man, always contented, and apt to break into song with a minimum of encouragement, his favourites being "Swanee" and "Old Man River". He beamed at the grandchildren, his daughter and anyone else around, especially if he had a full glass

177

of beer in his hand, but beer as a commodity had to be rationed to Grandpa.

Grandpa thought he was still with the Santa Fe, and did not realise that he was in Japan. Shortly after arriving in Japan, he saw a lot of Japanese walking past the house.

"There are a lot of Indians walking about here today," he remarked to his daughter. He soon came to accept the fact that there had been a sudden phenomenal increase in the population of Red Indians. On another occasion, when travelling to Kariuzawa, he looked out of the train window at the Kariuzawa river, rather a miserable stream. "By God," he said, "the Colorado River is mighty low this year." Preoccupied with railroads, Grandpa at first caused consternation at Shinjuku Railway Station by appearing at the ticket window, flashing his Santa Fe pass and demanding a free ticket to Chicago. Gradually the station employees came to know him and would issue a return ticket to the first station up the line. The station master there, forewarned from Shinjuku, eased Grandpa out of his carriage and onto a return train.

Sometimes Grandpa would wander and get lost. Eventually the military police would pick him up and he soon became a well-known figure. As Bill was known to be close to MacArthur, they were only too glad to cooperate. But it was at Shinjuku on his beloved railway station that Grandpa finally met his downfall. While striding along the platform to board his train, Grandpa suddenly decided that some poor, innocent Japanese farmer, making one of his infrequent visits to the great city, was wearing his overcoat. He ordered the farmer to return the coat. The Japanese had hardly set foot in the metropolis before he was involved in a fracas with a city slicker and a *geijan* (foreigner) city slicker at that. He refused to part with his coat and Grandpa, incensed at the behaviour of the Red Indian, wrestled with him. Both fell to the platform, and were rescued and separated by the station staff. Grandpa's temper, seldom raised, continued to be displayed for some time, and all involved were whisked off to the military police headquarters where the incident was resolved to everyone's satisfaction except Grandpa's. A few days later Bill was informed that Grandpa getting lost or travelling on the Santa Fe Railroad was one thing, but creating an international incident was another, and regretfully Mr Bloom should arrange with the Army Transportation Section for Grandpa to be returned without delay to ZI. This term baffled me for several months after my arrival in Japan but eventually I found out It meant Zone Interior, which is how the American Army were apt to refer to the continental existence of the United States.

Douglas MacArthur was a great Supreme Commander in his capacity as the ruler of Japan, and it is this aspect of his life which should become most honoured.

Although no doubt a brilliant general, he exercised his authority with an autocratic hand as though it was his by more than mortal dispensation. When he arrived in Australia during early 1942 to take over all the Allied effort in the Pacific, one observer noted that it was more like the Roman proconsul coming to take over his province than a general coming to an ally in distress.

One of the reasons why the numerous allies under MacArthur did not protest at his dismissal was that he had never during World War II nor in Korea mentioned the identity of any of the Allies. In his reports he would mention units of the American forces but he lumped together the fighting and endeavours of others under the indiscriminate term Allies. The Allies resented this, and his imperious attitude.

The British forces in Korea gradually built up a strength of 60,000 including the Army, Air Force and Navy. These figures were recorded in a letter from General Sir Anthony Farrar-Hockley. He was Adjutant of the 1st Battalion of the Gloucesters, at the time when they fought an epic battle in April 1951 in Korea. The General should know the figures as he is writing the official history of the Korean War for the Ministry of Defence.

When General Matthew B. Ridgway took over command of all land forces in Korea, morale was at a very low ebb and as he says in his *The War in Korea*:

"There was a loss of confidence and lack of spirit. Information was provided glumly, without the alertness of men whose spirits are high. I could not help contrasting their attitudes to that of a young British subaltern who had trotted down off a knoll to greet me when he spotted the insignia on my jeep. He saluted smartly and identified himself. Knowing that the British Brigade had hardly more than a handful of men to cover a wider sector of the front line, with a new Chinese offensive expected almost hourly, I asked him how he found the situation.

" 'Quite all right, Sir' he replied quickly. Then he added

with a pleasant smile: 'It is a bit draughty up here.' "

In April 1951, General Farrar-Hockley was a Captain with the Gloucesters stationed on hill 234. The Chinese attacked in overwhelming numbers just before midnight on the 22nd April. The attacks continued day and night, coming on in reckless waves. Neighbouring regiments, the Northumberland Fusiliers, the Royal Ulster Rifles and a Belgian battalion, conducted fighting retreats under appalling fire but the Gloucesters were surrounded. Relief columns were driven back; supply by air continued until the perimeter was so small that the drops fell into Chinese hands. The survivors were completely exhausted by mid-day on the 26th when the final distribution of ammunition was made. One and a half magazines for each Bren gun, three rounds per man still able to bear arms, and seven grenades between the whole force. When every round had been fired the remnant of the battalion started to try to escape, a hopeless endeavour.

It happened two weeks after MacArthur's recall. One wonders if he would have deemed this epic worthy of inclusion in a despatch. He certainly did not mention it in his memoirs.

MacArthur's egotism and iron will, his menace as a potential Republican candidate opponent to President Truman, his frequently expressed scorn of both Truman and before that Roosevelt, and his almost autonomous running of the Korean War, raised visions again of a general of the Roman Empire returning to take over the homeland at the head of his victorious legions. President Truman was a small man, but only in size. His heart was big and his resolution matched that of MacArthur. He summarily dismissed MacArthur.

The sudden inglorious exit of MacArthur and his weakness as an Allied commander should not detract from an achievement which is lasting and magnificent. His rule in Japan was masterful. The foundations of the Japanese-American alliance were laid by him.

MacArthur's power was enhanced by his showmanship; his full austere figure moved across the scene with military smartness and gravity. He always wore his uniform, surrounded by the soldiers of his guard — his Practorian Guard — all tall men with their white helmets adding to their stature. He was a master figure, all powerful but just, and the Japanese were surprised at first. Soon they came to have a deep respect and boundless admiration for the man.

MacArthur was able to conduct his affairs with extra efficiency because all his staff — from the humblest soldiers in his honour guard up through the ranks of the lower orders to the top civilians and military men - - were MacArthur men. Dissenters got short shrift, finding themselves rapidly returned to ZI (there it is again). There may have been a few who were not in his band of believers; if so, they kept their mouths shut. I never met a single one. Even non-Americans had to be careful, as a few foreign news correspondents found to their sorrow. They were out of the country in twenty-four hours, escorted to the airport by a few burly military police.

So, when the small man went from Washington to Hawaii to see the great commander and then dismissed him, the Americans in Japan and the Japanese were stunned. The effect on them was similar to being struck by lightning. I particularly remember Tom Gentry, whom few would call a sentimental man, saying, "It is as though my father had suddenly died."

The farewell in Japan was typical of the man: a tremendous show. Two million Japanese lined the route from his residence to the airport, troops marched, bands played, the air war in Korea halted as squadrons of bombers and fighters roared overhead. The stern figure sat alone in his car gazing rigidly ahead as it slowly moved through the city streets to Haneda Airport. The Japanese crowds bowed as the car went past. The exit was as glorious as the arrival.

There was only one Japanese who could steal the show from MacArthur. Promptly every day at 4.00 p.m. MacArthur would emerge from his headquarters in the Dai-Ichi Building in downtown Tokyo opposite the park around the Emperor's Palace. Impeccable in his uniform he would pause and gaze over the heads of the crowd who always assembled. His guards snapped to attention, moving with perfect drill, and saluted. He descended the steps, got into his long black limousine and hurtled off the half mile to his embassy residence through streets cleared of traffic, with military police on motorcycles as outriders. It was impressive, precise and brief; everyone liked it. But the man who stole the show was the small Japanese traffic policeman mounted on a dais on the street intersection outside the Dai-Ichi Building. He brought the traffic to a halt, with his tiny figure in police blue, white sleeved arms, white baton, and whistle in mouth. He would turn like a marionette, jerk his arms with fantastic speed, wave his baton like a flailing piston, and blow his whistle with a piercing note. This went on for two or three minutes till the traffic was halted when suddenly he would freeze, the burst of energy stopped as though the world had stopped. Fifteen seconds later MacArthur appeared at the top of the steps. It was worth seeing MacArthur's daily departure from HQ but quite a number of people turned up more than once to watch the traffic cop.

Chapter 24

SURGERY IN SECRECY

Hal and his tall tales — A saving song in the jungle — Mistaken nationality — A tricky piece of surgery — Improving a bad elbow swing — An unsolved mystery.

The question is often asked of me if there is a difference between treating Orientals and Westerners. The answer is that there is not, when it comes to operating anyway. Of course, the disease pattern is slightly altered. There are certain conditions, ulcerative colitis for one, which are practically unknown in the Chinese and Japanese; in a Caucasian a mass in the liver is likely to be a secondary growth from an intestinal tumour whereas in an Oriental, it is very likely to be a primary liver tumour. A torn cartilage in the knee is almost unheard of in Orientals, for the simple reason that the knee cartilage is either absent or so small that it does not get caught between the bones of the knee and torn in the thrusting movement, which is particularly common in football and other forms of sport. Enlargement of the prostate gland is much less prevalent in the East, although some surgeons argue that fewer men reach the age of sixty.

What the Oriental loses on the swings he makes up on the roundabouts, as he is subject to a higher rate of some organic diseases, as opposed to infectious diseases, than the Occidental. For instance, bleeding from a duodenal ulcer with few warning symptoms occurs frequently in young men in the East. But by and large the problems of surgery are the same in the East or West. You deal with them in the same way, although with all generalisations there are exceptions; the most notable in my experience being the treatment of duodenal ulcers. In the West the pendulum has swung in favour of dividing the vagus nerves to cut down the excretion of the stomach acid, one of the potent factors in causing an ulcer. Most Chinese surgeons still remove the ulcer because the two long-term complications do not occur in Chinese and Japanese.

One's reputation as a surgeon is often influenced by good or bad fortune and gratitude is seldom accurately linked to the difficulty of the problem. The successful completion of a long and technically difficult case gives a surgeon great satisfaction, and he is faintly surprised when the patient seems to consider the matter as almost routine. On other occasions the patient is absurdly grateful for what is a simple standard procedure.

One day, the senior man in a large British firm in Japan came to see me with haemorrhoids, or piles. The condition was far too advanced for any treatment except an operation but he dreaded the idea. He had spoken to friends who told him of their appalling experiences with pain and discomfort. He refused the operation, and the haemorrhoids were injected. This treatment worked very well and he was immensely pleased but, exactly as I had warned him, back they came in a few weeks. We tried another injection. There was a spell of temporary improvement of shorter duration and finally, in a state of almost abject terror, he entered the Bluff Hospital in Yokohama for operation. At that time spinal anaesthesia was used commonly. The orders left for pain-killing drugs were precise and liberal. The next morning on seeing me, he greeted me with, "The anaesthetic has not worn off yet." A horrible thought flashed through my mind, that of permanent paralysis. This I had never seen but it has been known to occur, probably due to the spinal needle puncturing a blood vessel with bleeding into the spinal canal. In a moment of panic I whipped down the bed clothes and pinched his thigh.

"Ouch!" he said, "what the devil are you doing?" He became the big business tycoon instantly, and a young man was taking unwarranted liberties.

"You felt that?" I asked.

"I certainly did."

"Well, the anaesthetic has worn off, that is evident. If it had not it could have been serious."

"It must be acting, I have no pain or discomfort at all; in fact I would not really know that I had been operated upon," he replied.

"I am afraid that the discomfort will come," I replied, but I was wrong. At no time did he have any pain or discomfort at all. I think he told the whole foreign population of Yokohama how marvellous I was. No amount of telling him that it was a colossal stroke of good luck had any influence. He was convinced that I was a genius and broadcast his opinion.

The British firm of which he was the manager seemed to specialize in giving me mental shocks. One of its younger recruits was Hal, who lasted longer with the firm than was warranted because he was not only inefficient and lazy, but a born liar. Hal was variously a renowned pilot in the Royal Navy, a bomber pilot in the RAF, a tank commander in the Western desert, a commando, a secret agent dropped into Yugoslavia; his war service changed according to his audience. He was certainly a thorn in the flesh of Findlay Cessford, his immediate superior in the shipping side of the firm.

Towards the end of his career with the firm, Hal was involved in a nasty car accident and landed up in the Bluff Hospital with a fracture of his leg. The fracture was not one which caused displacement of the bone fragments, but the fracture line did run into and involve the knee joint. After applying a full leg plaster cast I chatted to Hal and told him he was lucky that his injury was not severe, but that one always had to be a bit cautious in making predictions when a fracture involved a joint surface. I returned to Tokyo.

The next day Findlay Cessford appeared in my office.

"You know I can't stand Hal," he said, "but still I would not wish this on my worst enemy. I saw him this morning."

"Oh, I don't know," I replied, "it is not all that bad after all."

Findlay gave me a queer look.

"Really, Gren, I know that surgeons tend to take nasty situations in their stride, but after all Hal is a young man and the loss of a leg! Well, I must say I think you are a bit callous."

It was my turn to exhibit a startled look. I immediately thought that after the plaster had been put on, the leg had become so swollen in the rigid confinement of the cast that it had stopped the circulation and that the toes protruding from the end of the plaster had become gangrenous overnight — a surgeon's nightmare.

"Was Dr Morton there?" I quickly asked Findlay. "Has he not taken the plaster off?"

"No."

"You mean, no he was not there, or no he has not taken the plaster off?"

"He was not there."

We stared at each other for a few seconds.

"Well, who thinks the leg needs to be amputated?"

"You do," said Findlay in exasperation.

"I do?"

"Yes, you do."

"Who told you?"

"Hal told me this morning!" he said.

"Was he in pain?"

"No, he seemed quite comfortable."

"Look, Findlay," I replied, "we all know Hal is a monumental liar. I told him that the fracture was not severe or displaced but because it does run into the knee joint one has to be a bit more careful. This is all I said and the word amputation was never mentioned, or even considered. I thought when you spoke to me just now that the foot had become gangrenous due to too tight a plaster cast. You nearly gave me sudden heart failure."

"The damn son of a bitch!" yelled Findlay. "He was lying there with tears running down his cheeks. He said that you had told him that there was at best a ten per cent chance of saving his leg. I am sorry I called you callous. I must say I thought it was a bit unlike you."

Subsequently quite a few people — mostly good-looking girls — congratulated me on saving Hal's leg!

Whether this incident was material in Hal's departure from the firm in a hale and hearty state with both legs still firmly attached is problematical, but the break came a month or two later. As the date approached for Hal's departure Findlay started to upbraid his wife and their servant over the mysterious disappearance of articles of clothing. He was down to a bare minimum of shirts, socks, underpants, vests, handkerchiefs, and was also missing a sports jacket.

The Cessfords' flat was next to Hal's flat on top of the shipping office building.

"Darling," he said to his wife, Rene. "The washing is hung up at the back. I am damn sure Hal has swiped my things. I am going to go into his flat and search his baggage."

"You can't do that," said Rene, who was a gentle soul.

"I am damn well going to," Findlay retorted.

Suiting action to the word, Findlay marched across the hall, pressed the bell, pushed past the Japanese maid, and entered the bedroom where a trunk and suitcase lay packed but still open. He found five of his shirts, five pairs of socks, several vests and underpants, his sports jacket and one or two of his ties including his regimental tie. Finday did not see Hal off on the ship, as he was too busy sitting at home guarding his possessions.

I often dropped in at the Cessfords' flat on my way back from Yokohama. One day an incident occurred which has no relation to surgery but which has always stuck in my memory. While we were drinking a cup of coffee, the radio started to play the tune "Now is the hour when I must sail away".

"You know, Gren, that song saved me," said Findlay.

"How?" I asked.

"After the fall of Singapore," Findlay related, "I escaped with several soldiers in my company to Sumatra. We started walking south across the island to try to reach the south coast in the hope of getting a ship to Australia. We had to keep to the jungle trails in the hills to avoid the towns and villages, as the Japanese were already advancing across Sumatra and Java. After a few days we were completely out of food and very depressed. We stopped on a ridge looking down at a small town in the floor of the valley. The soldiers decided to give up and go down to the town to get food, despite the risk of capture. I tried to dissuade them, even ordered them, but to no avail and off they went leaving me to continue alone.

"I continued by myself, working my way southward by my compass along the tortuous jungle trails. I made little progress. When I looked down I could still see the lights of the town."

Hungry, dispirited, frightened and alone, his resolve began to waver. Should he also go down to the town? He lay down in the jungle hoping that his fortitude would be regained with the coming of dawn.

Suddenly, from quite close, he heard some voices singing "Now is the hour". He got up and made his way towards the singing to find a group of New Zealanders. They all starved together, but New Zealanders have a quiet resolution in both victory and adversity. Findlay and the New Zealanders made it to the coast to find a ship which took them to Ceylon. The soldiers who had descended to the valley were never heard of again.

Working mainly with Americans it is inevitable that you pick up something of their accent and it is simpler to use their expressions for the sake of clarity of understanding. Californians would sometimes think that my origins were in New England and this fact influenced another case.

Rainer worked for the Yokohama PX store. One morning, feeling off-colour because of a vague abdominal cramp, he went to an army hospital and was given some medicine. He reported sick within an hour of these symptoms but by evening was feeling a lot worse and went to the Bluff Hospital. It was Dr Morton who made the diagnosis of appendicitis and called me down to Yokohama.

Rainer subsequently sang my praises for diagnosing a ruptured appendicitis. All I did, in fact, was to confirm the diagnosis and operate. While everyone likes praise, honesty forced me to tell him that appendicitis is often very easy to diagnose when the classical picture has developed, but that several hours elapse before this stage is reached. Most people who develop appendicitis are not seen even by general practitioners before three or four hours at the earliest, and in the first hour when all he complained of was vague cramps and nausea without fever or right-sided abdominal pain, the diagnosis would be impossible.

Nothing would convince him of this. He had some hard words to say about the army hospital, and compared my skill with theirs to my great advantage. Later he sent me several other patients and also gave me a fine radio.

Rainer had a stormy time with peritonitis and a pelvic abscess and was in hospital for a month. At the time he was discharged I said to him, "You owe your life to a Scotsman."

"What do you mean?" he asked.

"Sir Alexander Fleming discovered penicillin and that is what saved you."

He was a bit shaken by this statement and asked for confirmation from Dr Morton. At that time Americans were apt to think that everything good originated from the USA.

Morton told me afterwards that he almost had to re-admit Rainer in a state of mental shock.

"Not only is Dr Wedderburn right about Fleming," he told him, "but you realise he himself is a Scotsman."

"Gee," said Rainer, reeling from the double blow. "I thought he came from Boston."

Dr Morton had the oportunity of surprising me not long afterwards. It all started when two men came into my office. Both sat down, but one got up at once to open the door and peer out. He was making sure that no one was listening. After some preamble he produced an X-ray of the thigh. Nestling beside the bone was the shadow of a bullet. His friend exposed his leg and showed the wound of entry.

Could this bullet be removed in secrecy, they wanted to know. It could, I said, but not in the office as finding a foreign body even as large as a revolver bullet can be quite a difficult job, and demands the facilities of an operating theatre.

How could secrecy be maintained, they asked. They would return the next day.

At the next visit I explained my plan Firstly, I pointed out that as one could not take a patient into the operating theatre and start making incisions in his leg without giving some sort of reason, I proposed to take a piece of beef bone, sterilise it, wrap it in sterile gauze, and put it inside the wrist of my operating glove. Furthermore, as an X-ray is a silhouette I would X-ray the leg or a leg — possibly my own — with the piece of bone underneath and the bone would appear to be in the leg. I would say it was a sequestrum, that is a bit of bone which detaches itself from the main bone as a result of infection. This would not fool a doctor, but I reckoned it would do for the nurses. The fact that there was an entrance wound could add to the story as it would seem to be the site of an abscess from the old infection. I went on to explain that, when I felt the bullet with my fingers, I would ask someone to bring the X-ray closer. While peering at the X-ray, I would lift the bullet out, push in the bit of bone, and then remove it in its turn in triumph for all to see. The bullet would be slipped into my glove or dropped on the floor and covered with my foot

It was about this time that I made a soft enquiry as to how the bullet got there. I knew already that they were members of the Counter Intelligence Corps. No answer was at first forthcoming. However at a subsequent interview there was some vague mention of a Russian submarine off the coast of Hokkaido, Japan's northerly island. This was a mere hint and my lips were sealed. The whole thing was so secret that even the army authorities should not know, so the army hospital was out of the question. I felt I was almost a member of the Secret Service myself.

In due course it all went as planned except for one moment of panic. Almost as soon as the incision had been made at the intended point, my fingers felt the bullet. When I knew it could be grasped and moved I asked for the X-ray. While it was being brought and everyone's attention directed at the X-ray picture, the bullet was removed, pushed into my glove with a conjurer's sleight of hand, and the piece of bone shoved in. The panic occurred when for a few seconds I could not relocate the beef bone.

I thought to myself, "Damn! I have the bullet out and now have lost the blasted beef bone." However, it was only a few seconds before I found it and pulled it out for an admiring audience. I retained the piece of bone, ostensibly to give to the patient. Actually, I did not want anyone looking at it too carefully. Both bone and bullet were given to Mr Smith. Honour was saved, deception had been perfect, and the cold war had advanced another step in favour of the Allies. I wondered if I deserved a medal.

The operation had been done as an added security measure when Dr Morton, the Superintendent, was away.

To my horror, some two weeks later Morton said to me, "I hear you took the bullet from Smith's leg."

"Yes, you seem to know I did — it was all supposed to be very secret."

"You bet it is secret."

"What about this Russian submarine business, do you know about that?" I asked.

"Good heavens, did they tell you that cock and bull story? They did not want to go to the US Army hospital because Jones accidentally shot his pal in the leg in their billet when he was fooling with his revolver. Everyone knows it would have been a court martial offence."

The British Naval Attaché at the Embassy was a Captain of the Royal Navy. He was full and robust, and his voice had a stentorian volume more suited, one felt, to the days of sail. He should have been in command of a seventy-four gun ship of the line at Trafalgar rather than filling a diplomatic post in Tokyo. The Captain was a keen golfer, handicap about five. He appeared in my office complaining of pain in the elbow which affected his golf swing. It was the wrong sport because he had tennis elbow.

An injection is now effective but this was in the days before cortisone. At that time treatment consisted of three choices: to rest the arm in a sling, which would not have appealed to the doughty Captain; to embark on a prolonged course of physiotherapy; or manipulation.

The aim of manipulation is to catch the sufferer unaware. By jerking the arm violently in the correct direction, the muscle insertion is torn off the bone. The origin then reattaches itself a few millimetres closer, the strain is relieved and the pain banished. That is the theory anyway. The patient is warned in gentle terms before this is done otherwise the doctor might end up on a charge of assault. It is a one shot deal. If you do not succeed at the first attempt, the patient will not let you try again. It does not always work.

The Captain agreed. I gripped his arm, made a few gentle movements to allay his fears, and let him relax the muscles before suddenly giving the forearm an almighty jerk. The roar he let out would have startled a midshipman at the masthead, and certainly startled several patients in the waiting room. I pressed some pills into his hand to cover the immediate discomfort and he departed, voicing his opinion of me for everyone to hear.

A few days of calm intervened and from time to time I wondered what was happening in the naval office at the Embassy, till the sound of his voice was heard booming through the door of my office. A wild hope surged through me that he might have toothache and want to see John Besford. The hope was shortlived. My nurse put her head round the door to say that the Captain was in a hurry, and could I please see him without him having to wait.

"All right," I said, "better get it over with, send him in."

He burst in and crashed into a chair.

"Do you know what has happened?" he asked.

"No," I replied, with mounting trepidation, fearing a dozen lashes or a sentence to be keel-hauled.

"Marvellous, boy, marvellous," he boomed. "I went round Koganei in sixty-nine, best score of my life, never done less than seventy-one before."

"Great," I replied, the relief flooding through me.

"If you can get that result from treating my bad elbow, how about having a go at my left good elbow? Might improve my game further."

"It would not do any good to a normal elbow."

"Too bad. Are you absolutely sure?"

"Absolutely."

"A million thanks. Must have you round for a gin," he barked and was off.

"The man is a genius," he yelled at my secretary on his way out. "Went round Koganei in sixty-nine." My secretary and the patients in the waiting room were completely mystified.

A surgeon working in Shanghai as the Communists approached and later in Tokyo at the height of the cold war sometimes becomes mildly involved in semi-secret matters. As students, we were taught the penalties of divulging facts given in confidence, but sometimes diplomats will spread information by leaking a secret to someone, in

191

the expectation of that person going right out and telling this supposed secret to all and sundry. There were occasions when it seemed obvious that I had been selected as the tool to do this very thing; whether it seemed to me of importance or not, sheer obstinacy would prevent me from breathing a word of it to anyone. They could spread their information through someone else. But now I relate an incident which intrigued me and one to which the answer has never been revealed. It is now so distant in time that no harm can come from telling the story.

A man came to my office and gave me the usual talk about the Free World, the Allies and the like. He told me that if I agreed, a member of the Russian Embassy from just across the road would come to the office with a fairly severe self-inflicted but apparently accidental wound. I was asked to put him in hospital, inform a telephone number and await instructions. If the Russian asked for asylum there was another number to call when, if possible, he would be picked up in the hospital car park. Failing the pick-up I should put the Russian in my car and take him to the address which would be divulged if I called a number and gave the code word.

Nothing happened for three weeks but then the Russian did turn up. It must have taken courage and determination to inflict the wound which also had the appearance of an accident. He readily agreed to go to hospital and the intermediary met me even before I paid my first visit to the hospital. There had been other patients from the Russian Embassy before, who were always accompanied by a companion. The two I had put in hospital had also had a relay of constant companions. For no apparent reason this man seemed to be allowed to stay unguarded for much of the time which was even more surprising as his English was fluent. We had several quite long discussions, partly based on what I had been told to say and ask.

I once made the mistake of using the expression "the Free World".

He smiled whimsically and said, "You know that what you call the Free World, we regard as the slave world."

I felt that while his wound was healing rapidly little progress was being made with his defection and suggested that I ask point blank if he wanted to change sides. However, the intermediary would not hear of this and asked me to arrange a meeting in a bar on the Ginza after discharging the patient. The only trouble was that the Russian refused the invitation. He returned to the Embassy and later, I believe, to Russia. I saw neither the Russian or the intermediary again.

There were a lot of unanswered questions. Why did he inflict the wound on himself? There is no doubt that he did it, because the wound was very recent, about fifteen minutes old, and it had been predicted some three weeks before.

Why was the usual guard absent? Knowing that I could enter the room to see him, why did the intermediary not do so? The hospital sister said the patient had not seen any visitors. It appeared on the surface anyway that the object of the exercise was defection, so why was I told not to ask him, when arrangements were on hand to whisk him away if he suggested it? Why did the Russian refuse the invitation to meet in the bar, which did seem unnecessarily complicated? None of these questions were answered but one fact stood out a mile — I had been told only about a tenth of the truth, if any, and only one thing was certain. My name was put on a number of files without any benefit to me at all. A week later an unknown person with a streak of decency left an unsigned message in an envelope at my office saying that it would be inadvisable for me to visit Russia even as a tourist for a long time.

Chapter 25

SCENERY AND SEX

A photographer's delight — Cherry blossom time — A variety of entertainment — A casual attitude about sex — Missed moments with Marilyn Monroe.

During the past century, going back to the days of sail, ships' passengers and crews bound for Yokohama would see Mount Fuji in her magnificence as they tacked or ran to make their landfall. Prints and pictures abound of sailing vessels moored in Yokohama and, if the pictures are to be believed, Fuji has undergone some remarkable changes in shape and position. Many of the artists must have based their paintings on seafarers' tales because, even allowing for artistic licence, they have taken great liberties with Fuji.

In some paintings the height of Fuji soars to rival Mount Everest. Others show it as a perfect cone, while some have moved it from its position fifteen miles inland bang onto the Yokohama waterfront. All these changes are not necessary. Fuji stands magnificent in its own right.

Yokohama was always the main port for passenger vessels arriving in Japan, and Fuji was the first sight the voyagers saw on arrival and the last on leaving. The mountain became the symbol of Japan for visitors, and for the Japanese, too, it exercises a profound effect, filling them with a sense of pride that borders on religious worship. Fuji is Japan.

Despite the majesty of the mountain, and the frequent glimpses of its serenity, it is extraordinarily difficult to photograph. As its circumference at the base is seventy-eight miles, the photographer has to be fairly far away to get it all in. If a good position is found to take a complete picture, the day will be cloudy. During many weekends in Hakone National Park the snowcap would show above the hills around the lake. One would jump into the car, climb up the hills and emerge through the tunnel. There from an elevation of 5,000 feet Fuji lay in front but, in the short twenty minutes taken to do the journey, clouds would have rolled up to hide the summit partially or would have drifted across its flanks. In summertime the snow usually melts, completely diminishing the appeal.

Excellent photos are, of course, legion. Some men spend all their adult life photographing Fuji from every conceivable angle but the amateur is perverse and wants his own picture. A score of times my car was thrust up the hill and through the tunnel before I was rewarded by the perfect cloudless day. From the tunnel exit, the base is below, some ten miles away, and the whole mountain fills the field of vision, rising to its height of 12,388 feet.

Of course, Fuji is not all of Japan, which is a mountainous country; there is very little flat land, except in the Kanto plain around Tokyo and in the Kansai around Kobe and Osaka. The hills for the most part are not too steep; most of the land is undulating foothills with terraced paddy fields and vegetable plots on the floor of the valleys. The villages and small towns have little attraction. There is a complete lack of order. The wooden houses could be made attractive by a coat of paint or by coloured tiles on the roof, but both paint and colour are missing except for the shop signs and advertisements which are garish without any attempt at uniformity.

As Japan came late into the modern age, electricity is carried overhead alongside telephone lines. The poles lean drunkenly, and wires cross and crisscross the streets. The roads have no definite margin, just fading on to the shoulders, which in turn end in an undetermined fashion in the dust or mud around the houses. One village has little to distinguish itself from another. In the fifties Tokyo itself, apart from the area around the Imperial Palace with its moat and weeping willow trees, was an ugly city.

At that time the roads of Japan were appalling for an advanced nation; a hundred and fifty miles was the limit to which anyone would drive. If you wanted to go further than that you took a train. The so-called Tomei Highway linked Tokyo and Osaka, the two major cities, and although the modern "bullet trains" do three hundred and fifty miles in three hours, it took an intrepid driver to travel the Tomei Highway, and at least two days to accomplish, provided the springs of the car held up under the strain, or the sump of the engine was not cracked by a loose boulder. Villages and roads left a lot to be desired, but the hills and coast are unique. Every headland and small island, some hardly bigger than a rock, carried its quota of pine trees, and one would wonder how a pine tree could survive on such a meagre base. But survive they do, and nowhere else in the world is this scenery duplicated.

Even the annual cherry blossom fails to make Tokyo attractive except for a few brief days. Cherry blossom time occurs in late April and is a great annual event. The newspapers report the advent of the blossoms in the south on the island of Kyushu. Hiroshima is a day or two ahead of Osaka and Kyoto, the ancient capital, while Tokyo is two days behind Kyoto. An early spring or a long extended winter makes a difference of only a day or two to the date when the blossoms flourish.

The cherry tree does not bear cherries, being of a different genus. The blossoms are white with a faint pink tinge, and do form a pleasant sight along roads bordered by a succession of trees or in clusters in parks. Provided it does not rain, the blooms last for four days, ending in a carpet of flowers covering the ground beneath the trees. If it rains heavily, which it is apt to do, the blossoms fall almost as soon as they come out. More impressive to my taste is the occasional wild tree standing out white against the green of a forest on a hillside. The cherry blossom has a great effect on the Japanese. The matron of the hospital used to give the staff the day off to go "blossom viewing", "Otherwise we don't get any work from them for the next year."

Japanese girls and women go in troupes to the favoured spots, while the men go on a colossal spree, swarming into the country in vast numbers. However, as they start drinking beer in huge quantities, only a small percentage manage to reach the beauty spots. Some fall by the wayside, others get so happy that they settle for any bit of country well short of their goal.

One year, we went to a famous park in the country to view the blossom. A contingent some thousand strong from the Tasaki Iron and Steel Works Cultural Association had the same idea. They chartered a train from Yokohama to visit the park, and duly arrived at the station. Meanwhile another contingent, from the Kusikosabu Manufacturing Company Recreational Club, chartered a train to another station close by. The roads from these two stations intersected a few yards from the park. As both trains were due to arrive in the early afternoon, there was plenty of time for the holiday makers to assemble before lunch and set off afterwards. They fortified themselves from mid-morning and did not neglect to carry additional supplies of beer and *sake* onto the trains. By the time they arrived at their respective stations they were just capable of forming into a rough column and proceeding up the road toward the park. The leaders carried banners in one hand and a beer bottle in the other, but the majority carried beer in both hands. The columns lurched forward, shedding an occasional alcoholic casualty who subsided by the wayside. The heads of both columns arrived simultaneously at the intersection. The bowing of the column leaders was sufficient to unbalance some, while others were toppled by their jolly companions pressing from behind; the heads of the columns met and collapse became general. The rear of the columns pressed on, and a vast heap of bodies blocked the road. Some lay where they fell, others struggled to their feet to bow to friend and foe alike, only to be bowled over once again by their own companions or members of the other team. No one got annoyed, bodies piled up, and the field of the battle of Waterloo had nothing on the scene.

In the early evening a heavy rain storm brought down the blossoms. Most of the two contingents never got into the park, and never saw the blossoms. Never mind, the Tasaki Iron and Steel workers had a great time. There was a universal hangover the next day when the stragglers found their way back to base and, after all, there was always next year's cherry blossom to look forward to.

While Japan is famous for its scenery and the cherry blossoms, what is less well known is the stunning variety of entertainment. Bars vary from small one-room shacks scattered throughout the suburbs to plush establishments on the Ginza. Dance halls increase in luxury and cost the nearer to the centre they are situated. Nightclubs are legion and usually there is a lavish floor show. It might be a chorus of twenty or thirty girls, a conjuror, an acrobat, or two or three well-endowed girls wearing only the briefest of pants. With luck you get a combination of them all. The tourist will visit the well-known expensive clubs, which are geared to extract his dollars in large amounts in the shortest possible time, but residents and the Japanese know of many clubs where the shows are better, the pace more leisurely and the pocket dented in a milder fashion.

The best show of this kind is the *Takarazuka*. It is named after a place near Osaka where *Takarazuka* has its own theatre. The girls, subject to firm discipline and training, join *Takarazuka* as young girls. They undergo formal education as well as choreography. The competition to be accepted is keen and candidates must have some basic dancing or singing capabilities as well as good looks. They are usually in training for two or three years before they appear at their own theatre or the Imperial Theatre in Tokyo.

The show they put on is top quality light entertainment,

expensively costumed, with imaginative dancing and excellent singing. Lavishly staged, it does not have any counterpart elsewhere. All the performers are girls. If a scene needs a boy one of the girls takes the male part.

Moving slightly down the entertainment scale but with a different motif, is the show between films at the Kokusai Theatre. Few tourists see this show, which is surprising because it is well worth it. On the stage, which must be one of the largest in the world, there are about three hundred girls near the finale of the forty-minute show. The costumes of the hundred-odd who are performing the main dance in the centre are of one design. A second costume group make their entrance from the wings or pop out of trap doors, while others emerge from doors amongst the audience, climb out of the orchestra pit and start dancing too. A huge backdrop curtain slowly lowers itself in the rear, also bearing its quota of girls on ledges and platforms. You begin to wonder if the whole girl population of Japan is assembled there. Everywhere you look there are acres of girls.

We took our daughters to the show. Soon afterwards we were in New York where we were taken to Radio City to see the Rockettes. As Americans know, the Rockettes have a rigid drill, dance in complete unison, and are something of a national institution. After the show our hosts asked my second daughter Alexi how she liked them.

"Lovely!" she said, "but they are not as good as the Kokusai." This remark was greeted by a stunned silence.

On a different level altogether was the fifth floor of the Nichigeki Theatre where the show is unashamedly strip and risqué. There is usually a bedroom scene of very doubtful propriety, but the comics are very good, and the audience laughs as soon as they appear. They remain funny to look at, even though it is impossible to understand the language, although a guess as to what they are saying will not be too far wrong. As they are comedians, the action normally ends in ignominious failure to achieve the obvious. Despite considerable progress and encouragement from the girl, the bed collapses or the comic falls out of the window. It is good vulgar slapstick and not offensive. This is followed by a dance team, all topless. The theatre is small and intimate, and the stage circular, with edges which extend outwards into the audience. If you are in the front row you are right in the middle of it all. One period of half an hour is indelibly etched in my memory, when a twenty-strong all-girl rumba band, wearing brief pants and transparent skirts and nothing else, swayed on all sides of me as they played all the funny instruments used in a rumba. The topless state seemed ideally created to accompany the movements of the rumba. The music was not bad either.

The Japanese have their own attitude towards sex. There is little stigma attached to it. The girls are full of curiosity and may indulge in sex in the way a foreigner might try a candy. Just take a candy if one happens to be around, and if the box is empty — well, no matter.

A series of incidents happened to Mortimer Wilson. I often had lunch with him in our office building and never remember him discussing women; as he was not boastful in this connection the story gains more credence.

His business of selling to the US Forces Clubs often involved joining sergeants for drinks in a bar on the Ginza. The Ginza is what Piccadilly is to London and Times Square to New York. While he was having a beer, a waiter put a glass of whisky on the table. Mort told him to take it away, as he had not ordered it. When the sergeant left Mort sat on to fill in time, when another whisky arrived. The waiter pointed to a well-dressed Japanese woman sitting nearby. She smiled and bowed slightly, and Mort actually thought that they must have met somewhere, although because of her looks and style he felt it was unlikely that he would have forgotten her. He joined her, took her to dinner and then back to his apartment. As the first light of dawn showed through the window she asked Mort if he would drive her home to Kamakura, a resort town down the coast. Mort tried to find out who she was but she asked him to stop in a side lane in Kamakura. She thanked him then disappeared round a corner. Most intrigued, he followed her to see her enter a very large house. Upon enquiry at the local police box he got quite a shock; she was the wife of one of Japan's very top industrialists, a household name.

Mort telephoned her. She was not too surprised to hear from him, but told him that as he knew who she was it must be quite obvious to him that they could not meet again. She would like to but it was impossible. She had really enjoyed herself, she said, thanking him.

Mort said, and it is almost certainly correct, "You know, she just wondered what it would be like to go to bed with a foreigner. Her husband was away and she decided, probably after asking her friends, to go to a bar on the Ginza frequented by Americans. There she looked around and decided on me!"

A month or so later Mort came back to his apartment late in the evening. The apartment was one large room, but a partition with shelves and bookcase separated the living room from the bedroom. Mort sat down to read a magazine when he heard a sound from the bedroom. Grabbing a stout wooden ornament as a weapon, he stealthily crept to the end of the partition to peek past it. There a girl lay in his bed, smiling up at him.

"Who are you?" he asked.

"Oh, I am a friend of Mrs T. She said she had a good time with you and told me to come."

Mort looked at her, considered the matter and said, "Move over."

"Did you take her home?" I asked.

"No, I told her to get a taxi."

"Not very gallant, Mort. Are you seeing her again?"

"No," he said. "She was not as good as Mrs T."

Japanese girls are attractive and exercise a fatal fascination especially on visitors. I was able to help two English businessmen make some contacts with a Japanese company, and they asked me to dine with them at the Imperial Hotel. We met in the bar, and after a drink or two one asked me where we should dine. There was nothing wrong with the Imperial; in fact the grill put out about the best dinner in Tokyo. I assumed that we would go to the grill but this suggestion was met with a lukewarm response. I suggested various restaurants. They might like Japanese food; alternatively a patient of mine owned a fine Chinese restaurant just up the road. There was a marked lack of enthusiasm.

"Well, we could go to a nightclub," I said.

"Yes!" came their answer in unison in a fraction of a second.

"But we are much too early," I replied glancing at my watch.

"Are they open as early as this?"

"I suppose so. We could get a meal at one of the better ones."

"Let's go," they said.

We arrived and were the first guests at Ding How's. The orchestra had not even uncovered their instruments. We sat down at a table and I called for the menu. Sitting and standing around the walls were some hundred hostesses. I could see my friends eyeing this bevy with delight and excitement.

"Let's just order our dinner," I suggested.

At this point the head waiter arrived and, before we got down to ordering the food, he asked, "Would you like some girls?"

"Yes!" they replied, again in unison.

"Let me pick them," I said. By this time I had made a plan to dine at Ding How's and get us all to go to the Cherry Bar. Madam Cherry came from Kobe and most of the girls in the Cherry Bar, a rather plush establishment, also came from Kobe. The girls in the Cherry Bar were reckoned by foreigners to be tops, a connoisseur's collection.

I walked along their serried ranks selecting the three ugliest.

"Just let them sit beside us. Give them an orange juice. Don't start feeding them, they don't expect it."

The head waiter asked the girls if they would like dinner too, to which they, of course, immediately agreed. The long dinner wore on. The band cranked itself into action, and my friends both danced with their girls. I ignored mine.

As dinner ended one of the men turned to me, "You really know the Japanese well. These are three charming girls!"

I took myself off to the Cherry Bar alone. One of the two more or less spent the rest of his time in Tokyo at Ding How's and his secretary sent me a letter from England in which she said that her boss wished to thank me very sincerely for the excellent contacts I arranged for them, and that the success of their visit was largely due to my generous help. I am sure he enjoyed dictating it to some stern female secretary.

Another businessman from England was more enterprising, and found a girl himself. He was quite well-to-do, in fact owning a firm with a well-known brand name. He arrived with a letter of introduction and also asked my wife and me out for dinner. When we met at his hotel he introduced Susie. Susie, he explained, was helping him with his shopping. Apparently Susie did the bargaining and saved him a lot of money in the process. Although Susie was no doubt a good shopper, Jean and I considered that she had some other attributes as well.

His stay in Tokyo was to be brief as he was a passenger on a freighter for the return trip to the United Kingdom. We bade him goodbye and bon voyage, so I was a little surprised to meet him in the street some days later. Susie was with him, and he explained that he had not finished his shopping, so he could take the train to Kobe and catch the freighter there. We said goodbye again.

A week later he called me up, saying that he had flu. I visited him in his hotel. Susie was there, presumably bargaining for reduced prices on the hotel food. He would catch a plane to Hong Kong to pick up the freighter. We said goodbye.

He missed the freighter in Hong Kong; he missed it in Singapore; he missed it in Penang, Aden and Port Said.

He came to my office with Susie.

"I have come to say goodbye definitely this time."

"Where is the freighter now?" I asked.

"Getting close to Europe. Luckily it puts into Antwerp and I shall board it there. After all, my wife will meet me when the ship berths in London."

"Really?" was the only immediate comment I could think of.

"Is Susie still helping you shop?"

"Yes. She has been a very great help to me. It was a big stroke of luck when I met her in the bar the second day I was here."

As Susie did not speak a word of English, and our friend spoke no Japanese, the shopping negotiations must have been an interesting experience.

What might be described as the laissez-faire attitude of many Japanese women towards sex formed a background to life in Japan which worried many foreign wives, who kept a close eye on their husbands. On hearing that Jean was going back to the United Kingdom with the girls a month or two ahead of me, the wife of the Royal Air Force Attaché showed concern.

"What," she gushed, "and leave your husband in the house with the maids. I would not do that for an instant."

"You have not seen our maid," Jean replied after a moment of startled surprise. I forget her name, but the maid was certainly a very ugly and unattractive woman as well as being somewhat stupid. It never occurred to me that she might harbour any romantic notions. Having seen Jean and the girls leave I was back in my house. After dinner I walked down the corridor to collect something from the bedroom. The door of the girls' playroom was open and the light on; sitting on a chair under the light was the maid, wearing a bright red dress with abundant white lace at the neck, cuffs and skirt. Her face was made up with layers of white powder, and she had a violent red gash of lipstick around her mouth. She looked like a caricature of Queen Elizabeth the First considering the advantages of executing

Mary Queen of Scots. For a second I was brought up short as she bestowed on me a sickly smile, presumably indicating welcome. I hurried on to the bedroom. Not wanting to go past the room again I went into the garden, got into my car and went off to a bar for a drink to restore my equilibrium, later to return back through the garden to avoid another confrontation. I did worry slightly; having spurned her unspoken offer, she might resign, which would involve me in the trouble of finding someone else.

I woke with the dawn, wondering what would happen. Promptly at seven she knocked, came in with the tray bearing the morning tea, and pulled back the blinds. Dressed in her uniform, worn in its customary sloppy fashion, she said good morning and went out. No glance, word or action subsequently seemed to relate to the night before. It might never have happened. I did not see the dress again, and the incident lasting possibly two seconds was like a brief but vividly remembered bad dream.

The affair of Lew Stone and his maid was much more protracted. Lew and his wife were sitting up in bed one Sunday morning reading the newspapers. Their small daughter came in to remark that she did not know that the chauffeur and the maid were married; she had found them in bed together.

Lew was sent down to investigate. The evidence was no longer available, but after some difference of opinion on how the matter should be dealt with, Lew and his wife decided to ask the advice of his company's Japanese adviser. They felt that the moral aspect should be considered. Lew was a member of one of the large oil companies and the adviser, a former member of the Japanese cabinet before the war, was a widely respected man of impeccable character; a gentleman to his fingertips.

"You must sack the chauffeur," was his advice.

Lew accepted this verdict but on reflection he was reluctant to lose the services of an excellent chauffeur, and his wife was reluctant to lose a very good maid. It was decided to approach the adviser again the next day to find out why dismissal was necessary. Would not a severe rebuke meet the occasion?

The next day Lew again asked the venerable Japanese why dismissal was necessary. The adviser looked at Lew with a surprised expression.

"The driver did not ask you if he could sleep with the maid," he said.

"I know he did not," said Lew.

"But she is your maid."

"I know, what difference does that make?"

The adviser's look turned to one of pained surprise. How could Lew be so ignorant? He decided to spell it out in blunt terms to this ignorant foreigner.

"You are the master. If anyone sleeps with the maid it should be you; it is your right. The driver should have asked you first."

Lew had lost face; the driver had usurped the master's privilege.

As there are several references to the girls and women in this chapter, it is appropriate that I mention my encounter with Marilyn Monroe. She was at that time married to Joe DiMaggio, the long-time star of the New York Yankees Baseball Team. Joe was friendly with Mr and Mrs Duddy, the manager of the Chase Bank in Toyko, and both Marilyn and Joe had been invited to dinner with the Duddys.

In the vast sprawl of Tokyo, the Duddy home was one of the nearest to ours, being a mere four minutes away. On the evening in question I was home and readily available, just a phone call away. When Marilyn and Joe showed up for dinner, she complained of feeling ill, and when her temperature was taken it was found to be 103°. Mrs Duddy suggested that Marilyn go to bed in the spare room and she and her husband agreed to call me to come round. Mrs Duddy was sure that I would not mind. She was dead right, I would have been round like a shot from a gun. Just before calling on the phone Mrs Duddy went into the bedroom to find Marilyn in bed with her clothes off.

"I will lend you a nightdress, dear," she said.

"No, thank you," replied Marilyn, "I never wear a nightie."

Mrs Duddy digested this remark and returned for a hurried consultation with her husband; she was somewhat straightlaced and the gist of their conversation was that she thought that Dr Wedderburn would be embarrassed to see Marilyn without her clothes, despite the fact that she was demurely tucked up under the sheets. Jim, a man more after my heart, expressed his opinion that I would be able to cope, but deferred to her opinion. They decided to give Marilyn a couple of aspirins and await developments.

If I had remained in blissful ignorance of this sinister decision all would have been well, but one of the dinner guests told me about it the next day when Marilyn's temperature had returned to normal. It was with some difficulty that I was civil to Mrs Duddy when we next met.

Chapter 26

SAYONARA

Entertaining visitors — Kabuki and Noh — The nightclub addicts —
An invitation to Hong Kong — The undiplomatic diplomat.

Throughout our five years in Japan we had a succession of visitors, most of them from Hong Kong. Usually they would stay for a few days to a week. It was an easy duty to entertain most of them, especially if they allowed us to do the planning. Others had preconceived ideas which they wished to fulfil. This suited me admirably provided that my presence was not always required.

Visitors interested in scenery were easy. In fact we saw several places and parts of Japan only once and that was when taking our visitors on a two- or three-day trip. Five Lakes on the remote side of Mount Fuji was one delightful place we saw with a doctor and his wife; many years later he took us on a three-day jaunt in Rhodesia which included the Victoria Falls.

Jean and I carefully planned such trips so that we ourselves would benefit from the new sights and scenery. It was hard, however, to avoid the well-worn spots of conventional viewing which usually included a temple. I must by now have looked at a vast number of temples all over the Far East. There is always a mild interest in looking at the main god who sits in the centre and is seldom less than twenty feet in height. He may wear a rather ferocious expression, especially in Chinese temples. If on the other hand he is Buddha, his expression is more benign as he gazes over the heads of those below with complete lack of interest. The bright colours in the background, the smell of incense, the odd monk or acolyte flitting about in the background on some obscure business is repeated. In Bangkok there is one temple with a difference. This is the temple of the Reclining Buddha, where he is lying on his side. It is quite a sharp walk from the feet until you reach the head, but his expression when you get there is of the same lack of interest. I tried to avoid temples or confine the time to ten minutes, not always with success.

Culture buffs were all right unless one got too involved. One couple expressed surprise that I had never been to the *Noh* Play; as a matter of fact, I don't think up to that time I even knew of its existence. *Kabuki* was enough for me.

Kabuki is traditional Japanese opera which flourishes in its own theatre. Even if you manage to get your hands on an outline of the plot printed in English the whole thing can be baffling. Every now and then some character may come on briefly to make a gesture which to the initiated means five years have passed since the previous scene, but you are left in the dark. Things go wrong too with the action. By close study you realise that the hero is fed up with his wife, probably on account of infidelity though she may be merely trying to do him down financially. This point may never be cleared up.

After working himself up over several scenes in half an hour, like a combination of Hamlet doing the worrying and Henry the Fifth exhorting his troops before the battle of Agincourt, the hero takes action by creeping into his wife's bedroom and decapitating her with a large sword. But there the trouble begins because the hero's girlfriend has chosen that night to occupy the wife's bed. Whether this is by caprice, accident or by skilled management on the part of the wife remains a mystery. As likely as not the hero may then despatch himself, but on the other hand, he may not. Of course, everyone is dressed in wonderful colourful costumes and an orchestra bangs away on drums and stringed instruments, and one never knows quite when to expect the drummer to have a go at crashing and beating the living daylights out of the drums. This action seems to bear little relation to what is happening on stage. The whole performance lasts about four hours. There are no women, as the female parts are taken by men. You totter out into the streets of Tokyo bewildered, deafened and with the impression that you have been ridden over by a squadron of cavalry.

But the *Noh* Play is different. The *Noh* has its own theatre, a small compact hall with several rows of wooden chairs. The stage, raised two feet, confronts the rows and has a projection some fifteen feet across protruding into the audience. On the edge of this projection sits the orchestra, four men squatting in their grey kimonos. Two have an instrument with one or two strings which they twang irregularly, but all four make the most unbelievable sound from deep in their throats, a sound I have never heard produced by humans before or since. It is a sort of humming groan rising at intervals to a falsetto whine. This grotesque sound, which goes on throughout the whole performance, is weird and completely without beauty or melody.

SAYONARA

I forget what the first act of one and a half hours was about. Only three men took part and it was all mime. Dressed in long kimonos they would stand immobile, turn slowly, raise a leg slowly and put it down, face the other way and possibly jump two steps right. It did not seem to have any meaning or purpose, and the "orchestra" ground away. During the interval, sagging back against the wall in the corridor, I shakily lit a cigarette when my guest turned to me.

"Isn't it wonderful?" he said.

Jean stepped right across my front giving me a very wifely look which was about the only thing I understood all evening.

We returned to our seats where I gloomily looked at the programme. The play was over and now we were to see the Lion Dance, the April Dance, the Prince's Dance and the Fisherman's Dance. It would last a couple of hours, and I wondered if I could hold out.

Back came the orchestra into action once more and then the actors with huge scraggy wigs to get down to the Lion Dance. The same slow motion performance started up again. A surreptitious glance at my watch showed twenty minutes elapsed time, when I noticed that one of the men had picked up a long piece of bamboo pole. It seemed to me that one action might have conceivably been similar to a fishing rod cast. A wild hope surged through me; maybe they had got the order wrong, but at least we had finished with the Lion Dance. The orchestra got up and bowed, the actors bowed, the stage lights went out; somewhere along the line I had missed April and the Prince. It was all over. Worried about my total lack of cultural understanding. I mentioned this to Father Rogandorf, a German, the Professor of Philosophy at Sofia University, the Catholic University in Tokyo.

"Dr Wedderburn," he said, "before I came out to Tokyo in 1939, I spent a few months in Oxford, England. I was once asked to get up at half-past five in the morning to go out to a field some ten miles away to watch some folk doing a Morris dance. I did not go. The *Noh* Play is in the same category. Would you get up at 5.30 and bicycle ten miles to see Morris dancing in a meadow?"

The guests who were the biggest strain were the nightclub addicts. Liz and George Watson came up from Hong Kong, where, in 1955, there were no sophisticated nightclubs or anything remotely like them; it took one visit to the Queen Bee on their first night to establish the pattern. I had cancelled anything remotely connected with surgery during their visit but I still had to face up to the office. Most clubs in Tokyo closed down at two in the morning, but not the Golden Gate which the Watsons did not find out about till the third day. Thereafter we closed it down every night. I missed my guests at breakfast but they were ready to face the day at lunchtime and in great shape for the coming evening.

While we enjoyed our time in Japan, we did not want to spend our working life there, and by 1955 Corinna and Alexi were reaching the age when education was becoming important. They were at the Convent School in Tokyo. This is an excellent school, international in its teaching but with an American slant, as most pupils were Americans. While it is ideal that a child should have an international rather than a national outlook, in practice this handicaps a child when the child returns to his own country because the syllabus he has followed is different and, inevitably, there are gaps in his knowledge compared to his fellows.

Jean and I decided to think of making a move and Jean suggested I ask George if I might join their practice in Hong Kong.

"Why not ask him today?" Jean asked.

"I will ask him on the last evening," I replied.

After dinner while girding our loins, and mine were about exhausted, George suddenly said to me, "Gren, the partners asked me to find out if you would like to join us in Hong Kong."

Being offered a job is quite different from asking for one. My exhausted loins took on a new lease of life. "The Latin Quarter, the Queen Bee and the Golden Gate, here we come!" I said.

The aspect of my decision which was the most distressing one was the effect it would have on my partners Bernard and Derek. Both of them were upset, but men of their characters did not indulge in recrimination or criticism; I continued to work with them for another nine months in the closest harmony. They both told me that they understood, and that the welfare of my family had overruling priority. Derek is still in Tokyo and Bernard and Susan retired to live in Lausanne, Switzerland in 1970. We have seen each other many times over the years since 1955.

A few days before we left Tokyo we were at a cocktail party at the American Club. Johnny Johnson, the president of the First National City Bank in Japan, introduced me to a newcomer to Tokyo with the words. "I don't know why I am introducing the doctor to you, unless you fall ill in the next few days, as he is leaving to practise in Hong Kong."

"That is interesting," said the man, "but how are you going to be able to stand the British down there?"

"Oh," I replied, "I think I shall be able to manage all right."

The incident would have passed but for Johnny. Like Falstaff, Johnny's frame and paunch shook with laughter.

"Don't you realise," said Johnny, "that Wedderburn is British!"

The guest departed hurriedly.

"He won't sleep tonight, Gren," said Johnny. "He is a new man in our Embassy. Not a very diplomatic remark, was it?"

"Ili, Vernc," Johnny's voice boomed across the crowded room to the host. "Come and hear this."

A spate of phone calls followed in the next three days from Americans expressing their indignation and apologies. Some demanded the diplomat's name which in truth I had missed on the introduction.

A year later I heard that Johnny Johnson had been promoted to head of the Far Eastern Department at the head office of the First National City Bank in New York, and was expected to visit the branch in Hong Kong. A card inviting me to a cocktail party in his honour arrived on my desk, but on his first day in Hong Kong a patient's slip with his name on it was handed to me by the receptionist.

Johnny entered. I rose to walk across the room to shake his hand.

Johnny stopped inside the door, holding up his hand like a judge demanding silence.

"Gren," said Johnny, "don't ask me. I am just able to stand the Americans in New York!"

EPILOGUE

Both John Besford, the dentist, and Leo Pickles, Her Britannic Majesty's Consul General in Japan, were awarded the Order of the British Empire by Her Majesty the Queen in the Honours List of January, 1975, and Derek Fair received the OBE in 1977.

FINIS